This book is a synopsis

of the larger book,

"Understanding Diabetes,"

12th edition.

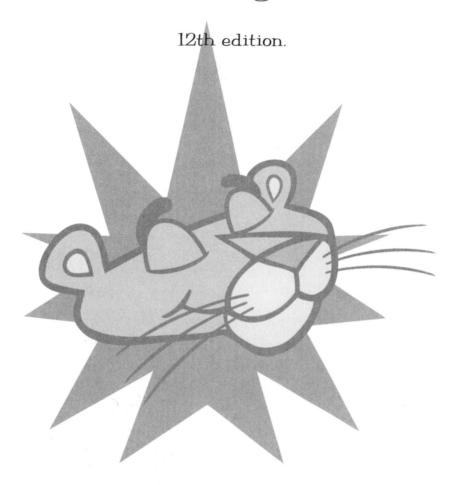

It provides a quick summary

of each of the 31 chapters.

It may be easier to begin

learning from this book

until you are ready

to read the larger book.

A First Book for UNDERSTANDING DIABETES

Companion to the 12th Edition of "Understanding Diabetes"

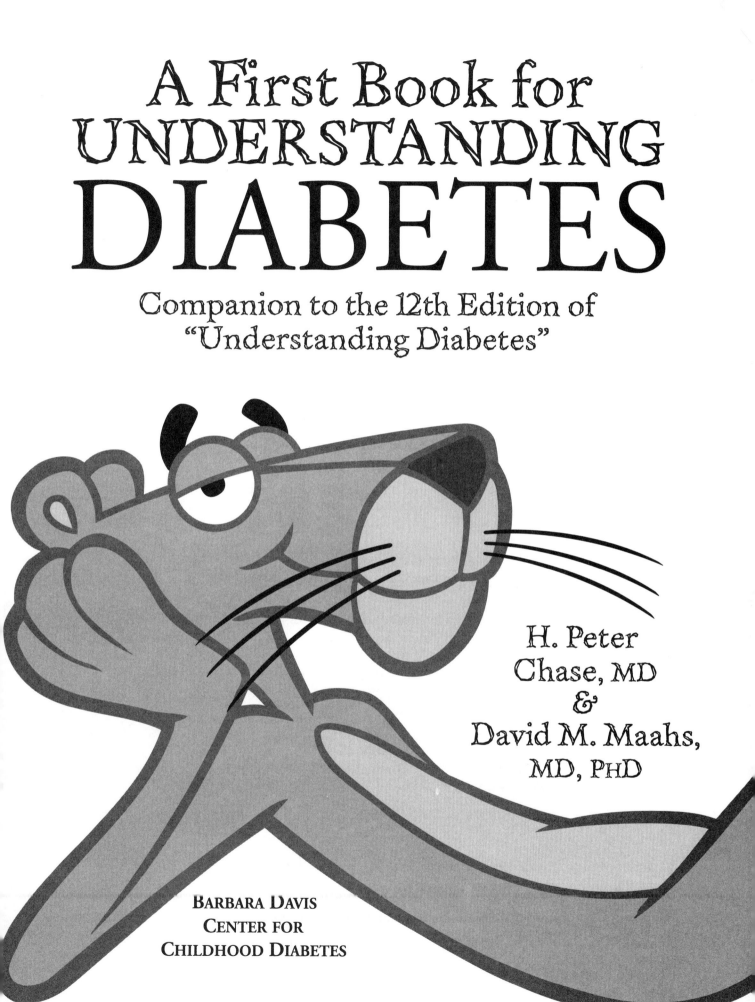

H. Peter
Chase, MD
&
David M. Maahs,
MD, PhD

BARBARA DAVIS
CENTER FOR
CHILDHOOD DIABETES

For information, contact

Children's Diabetes Foundation at Denver, Colorado
4380 South Syracuse Street, Suite 430
Denver, CO 80237

www.childrensdiabetesfdn.org

Chase, H. Peter.
    First book for understanding diabetes / H. Peter
Chase, David M. Maahs.
    p. cm.
    LCCN 2011929741
    ISBN-13: 978-0-983265016
    ISBN-10: 0-983265011

    1. Diabetes in children. 2. Diabetes.   I. Maahs,
David M. II. Title.

RJ420.D5C466 2011   618.92'462
                            QBI11-600118

Published by
Children's Diabetes Foundation at Denver, Colorado
4380 South Syracuse Street, Suite 430   Denver, CO 80237
303-863-1200

Book Design by Cindy Kalkofen

Printed in the United States of America
1 3 5 7 9 10 8 6 4 2

This book is dedicated to the
Juvenile Diabetes Research Foundation (JDRF).
Their support of research leading to the closed-loop (bionic)
pancreas will make life better for all people living with diabetes.

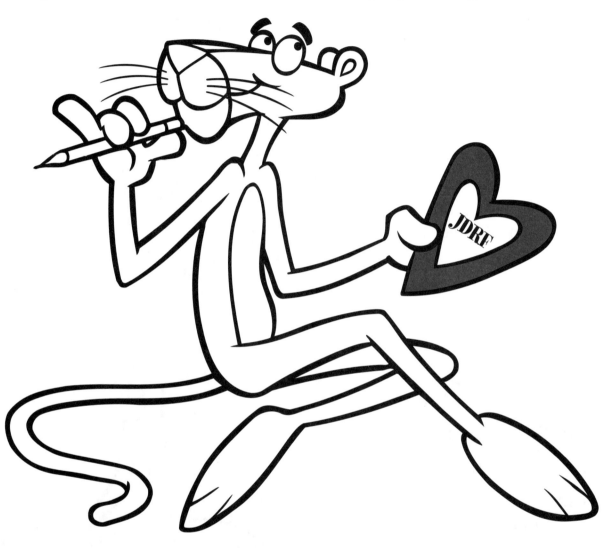

SPECIAL THANKS TO...

- The staff of the Children's Diabetes Foundation.

- Regina Reece for manuscript preparation, editing and proofreading.

- Cindy Kalkofen for book design, graphics, and illustrations.

- MGM Consumer Products for allowing the use of THE PINK PANTHER™.
  www.pinkpanther.com

- Additional copies of this publication may be purchased from the Children's
  Diabetes Foundation at Denver. See available publications at the end of this book.

Table of Contents

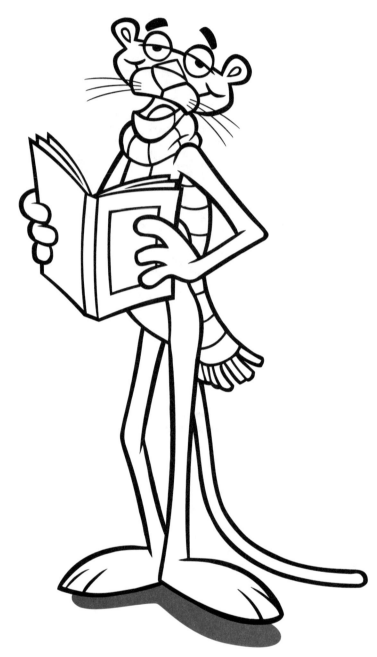

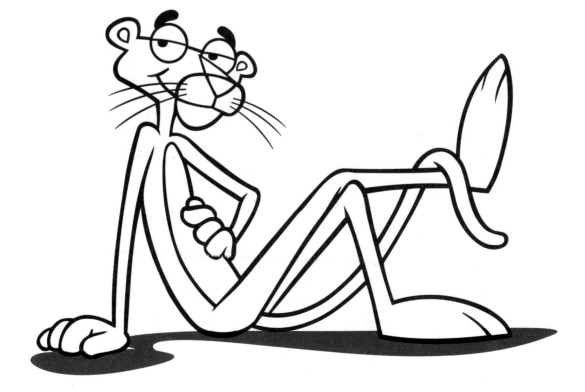

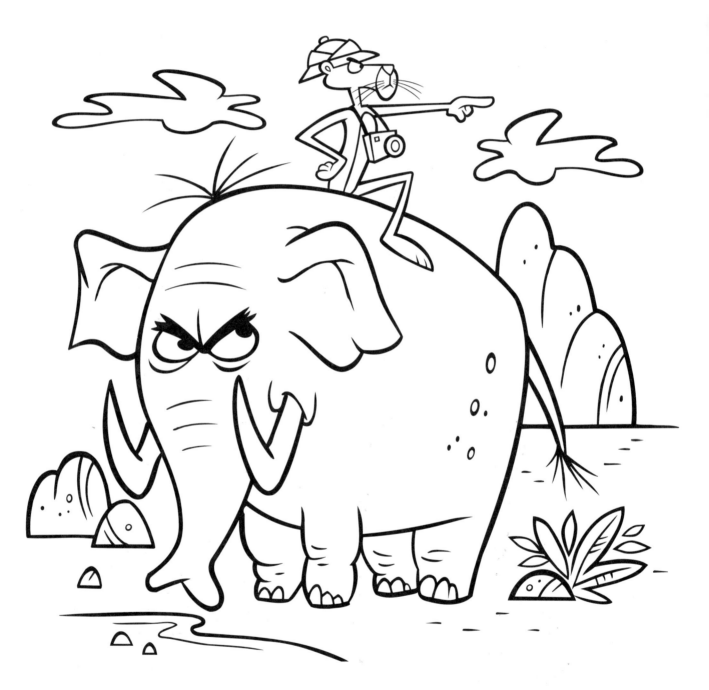

The Chapters in this book follow the chapters in "Understanding Diabetes," 12th edition.

Chapter 1
The Importance of Education in Diabetes

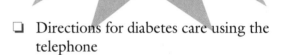

It is important to learn all about diabetes. At the time of diagnosis the family will spend one to three days learning about diabetes. A week later they will return for another day. This book will help in the beginning, until the family is ready to read the larger book, "Understanding Diabetes." In both books, the chapters have the same numbers and topics. All family members, including both parents, should be present for initial education. In this book we use "you" for you and your child.

Initial teaching (survival skills) often includes:

❏ What diabetes is and what causes it

❏ Urine and/or blood ketone checking

❏ Blood sugar checking

❏ Recognizing a low blood sugar and how to treat it

❏ Insulin types and actions

❏ Drawing up insulin

❏ Giving shots

❏ Food survival skills

In addition to survival skills, other areas often covered are:

❏ A school plan

❏ Directions for diabetes care using the telephone

❏ Details of treatment (including "thinking" scales)

❏ Education about food (dietitian)

❏ Feelings (psych-social team)

❏ Plans for the next few days

One-Week Follow Up

Usually at one-week the family and child return for group education with other families. The content includes teaching done by the dietitian and nurse and a clinic visit with the physician. Areas covered include:

❏ Details of food management with diabetes

❏ Review of HbA1c: what is it, why is it important

❏ Insulin actions and different insulin regimens

❏ Pattern management of blood sugars: how to identify trends and when to fax or email numbers (all families are given fax sheets to send in weekly for at least four to six weeks)

❏ Low blood sugar care: causes, signs and treatment of mild to severe low blood sugars including a review of the use of glucose tablets and gel and the administration of glucagon

❏ High blood sugar care: prevention of diabetic ketoacidosis; causes, signs and treatment

❏ Sick-day management: how often to check blood sugars and ketones, fluid replacement - what type and how much, when and how to urgently call for assistance.

The importance of education in diabetes.

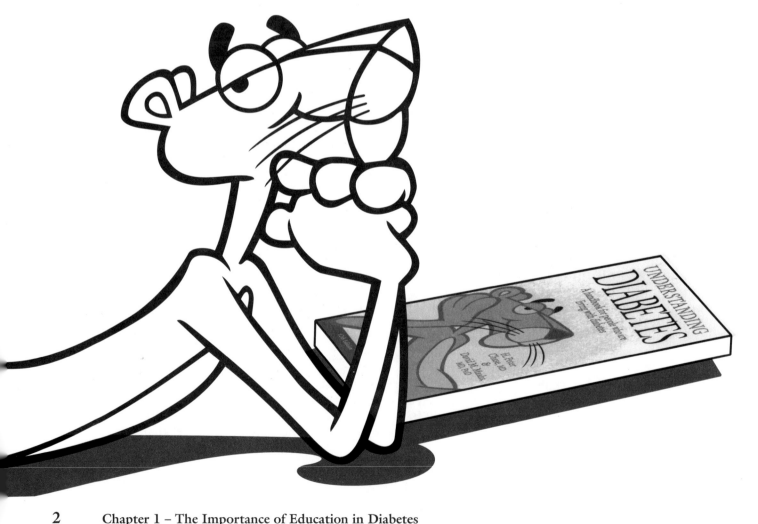

This is a general plan. The timing is varied and may change if the person is hospitalized versus when treated only in the clinic. A trend in recent years has been to teach survival skills in the first one to two days, and to make the visit at one week (when stress is lower) a longer and more in-depth visit.

New Patient First-Night Instructions for _____

A. *The diabetes supplies you will need the first night include* (*your nurse will mark which you need*):

_____ Blood glucose meter   _____ Meter test strips   _____ Alcohol swabs
_____ Ketone check strips   _____ Glucose gel & tabs   _____ Log book
_____ Insulin   _____ Syringes   _____ Phone contact card

The first night you will either get your insulin injection at our clinic, or you will give the shot at home or where you are staying.

B. *If the insulin is given while at the clinic:*

☐   1.   If rapid-acting insulin (Humalog®, NovoLog® or Apidra®) has been given, eat in 20 minutes if blood sugar is above 120 mg/dL (>6.7 mmol/L) (may need to eat sooner if below this level).

☐   2.   If regular insulin has been given, try to eat your meal within 30 minutes – or – have a snack containing carbohydrates on the way home if it will be more than 30 minutes (or if blood sugar is below 80 mg/dL [4.4 mmol/L]).

☐   3.   One of the above insulins and a longer-lasting insulin will be given to cover overnight insulin needs.

     4.   Allow your child to eat until their appetite is satisfied, avoiding high sugar foods (especially sugar drinks and sweet desserts).

C. *If the dinner insulin is to be given at home:*

1.   Check your child's blood sugar right before your meal. Enter the result into the log book.

2.   Check for urine ketones if directed. Enter the result into the log book.

3.   Call Dr. _____ at _____ or page at _____ for an insulin dose or if questions.

                     Give this dose: _____.

4.   Draw up and give the insulin injection right before your meal (see Chapter 9). If your child is not very hungry or is tired, you can give the shot after they eat and call the physician with any dose questions.

5.   Eat your meal, allowing your child to eat until their appetite is satisfied. Avoid high sugar foods.

D. *Before Bed:*

1.   Check your child's blood sugar. Enter the result into the log book.

2.   Check for urine ketones if directed. Enter the result into the log book.

3.   Call your physician at the numbers listed above if your child's blood sugar is below _____ or above _____, or if urine ketones are "moderate" or "large" or if blood ketones are >1.0 mmol/L. If urine ketones are "trace" or "small", have your child drink 8-12 oz of water before going to bed.

4.   Give an insulin injection if your physician instructs you to do so. (Dose, if ordered _____.)

5.   Have your child eat a bedtime snack. Some ideas for this snack include: cereal and milk, toast and peanut butter, a slice of pizza, yogurt and graham crackers or cheese and crackers. (See Chapter 12 in this book for other ideas.)

E. *The morning before coming to the clinic:*

1.   If your physician has instructed you to give the morning insulin at home before coming in, follow the steps listed above (see letter "**C**") and give dose as directed by MD before eating breakfast.

2.   If you have been instructed to wait to give the morning dose until after coming to the clinic, do a blood sugar test and a urine ketone test if directed upon awakening (if blood sugar is less than 70 mg/dL [<3.9 mmol/L], give 4–6 oz of juice promptly).
     Write the blood sugar and urine ketone results in your log book.

☐ Eat breakfast at home, and then come to the clinic for your insulin injection.
☐ Bring your breakfast to the clinic, and you will eat it after the insulin has been given.

3.   Please bring all blood testing supplies and materials you received the first day back to the clinic (including your log book, Pink Panther book, insulin and supplies).

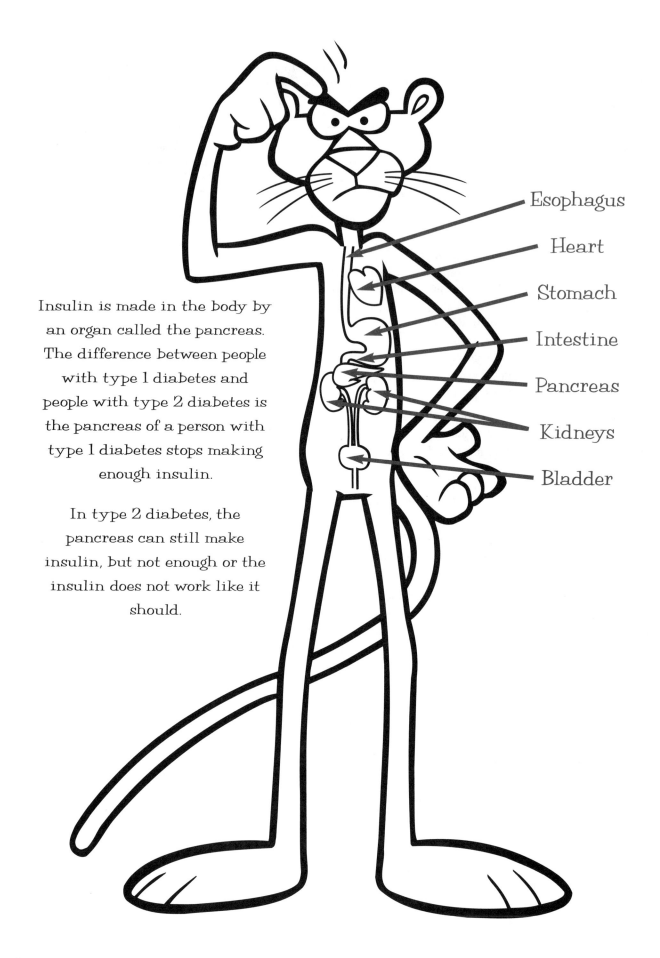

Insulin is made in the body by an organ called the pancreas. The difference between people with type 1 diabetes and people with type 2 diabetes is the pancreas of a person with type 1 diabetes stops making enough insulin.

In type 2 diabetes, the pancreas can still make insulin, but not enough or the insulin does not work like it should.

Esophagus

Heart

Stomach

Intestine

Pancreas

Kidneys

Bladder

Chapter 2
What is Diabetes?

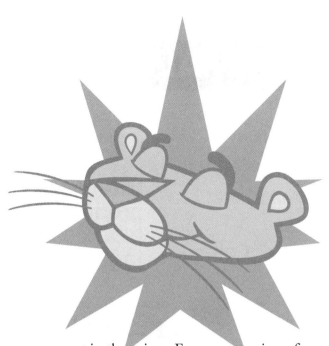

Type 1 (Childhood, Juvenile, Insulin-dependent) **diabetes** is due to not enough insulin being made in the pancreas (see picture). The most common signs are:

🐾 **frequent passing of urine**

🐾 **constant thirst**

🐾 **weight loss**

For people with **type 1 diabetes**, insulin must be taken through a needle. Insulin cannot be taken as a pill because the stomach acid would destroy it.

Type 2 diabetes (Adult-onset, or Non-insulin dependent diabetes) is different from type 1 diabetes. Insulin is still made but not enough, or it doesn't work very well. People with type 2 diabetes can sometimes use pills (which are not insulin) and diet and exercise to control their diabetes (see Chapter 4). Eating healthy food and exercising are also important for people with type 1 diabetes, but they will always need to take insulin shots.

Insulin allows sugar to pass into our cells to be used for energy. It also turns off the body's making of sugar. When not enough insulin is present, the sugar cannot pass into the body's cells. The sugar is high in the blood and it passes out in the urine. Frequent passing of urine is the result. (See Figures on the next 2 pages.)

Because sugar cannot be used for energy without insulin, the body breaks down fat for energy. Ketones are the result of using fat for energy.

When insulin treatment begins, the urine/blood ketones gradually disappear (see Chapter 5). After a few days, the blood sugars come into range and the excess passing of urine and drinking of water will decrease. Weight is gained back, the appetite decreases and the person starts to feel much better.

Often a **"honeymoon"** time begins a few weeks or months after a person with type 1 diabetes starts insulin shots. The insulin dose may go down and it may seem like the person does not have diabetes, but **THEY DO!** This period may last from a few weeks to a few years.

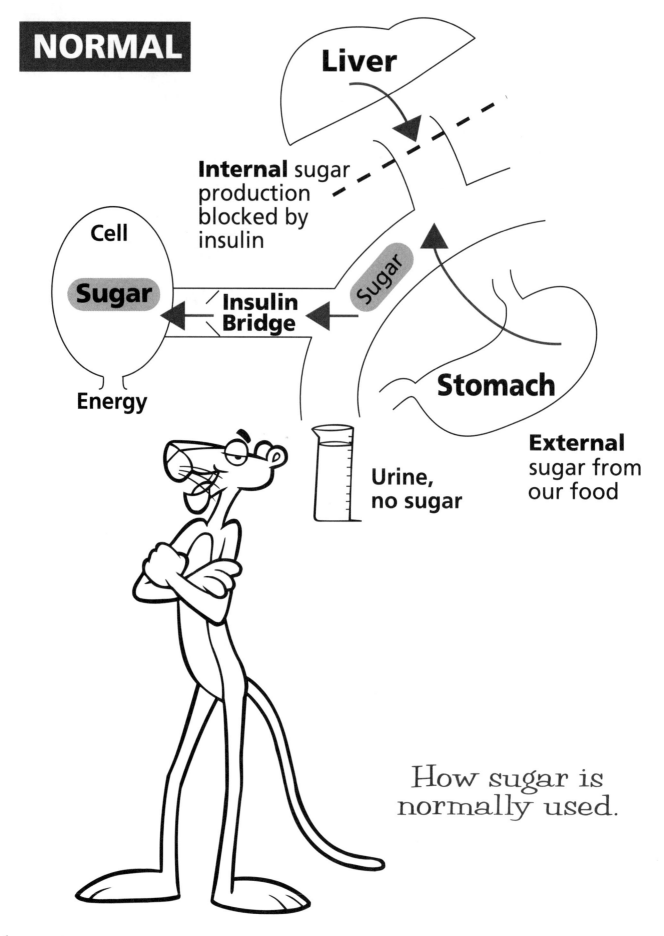

NORMAL

Liver

Internal sugar production blocked by insulin

Cell

Sugar

Energy

Insulin Bridge

Sugar

Stomach

Urine, no sugar

External sugar from our food

How sugar is normally used.

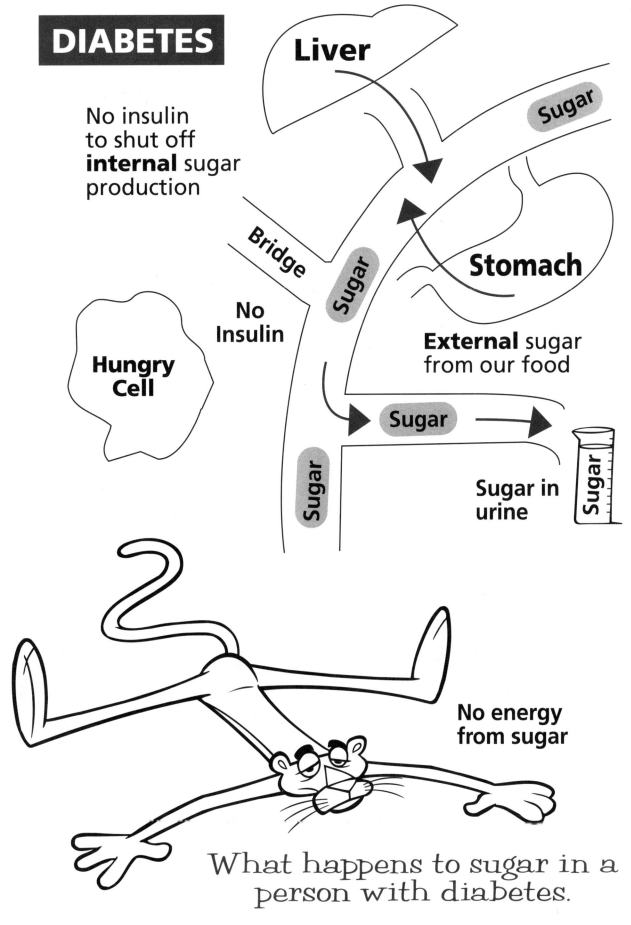

DIABETES

Liver

No insulin to shut off **internal** sugar production

Sugar

Bridge

Sugar

Stomach

No Insulin

Hungry Cell

External sugar from our food

Sugar

Sugar

Sugar in urine

Sugar

No energy from sugar

What happens to sugar in a person with diabetes.

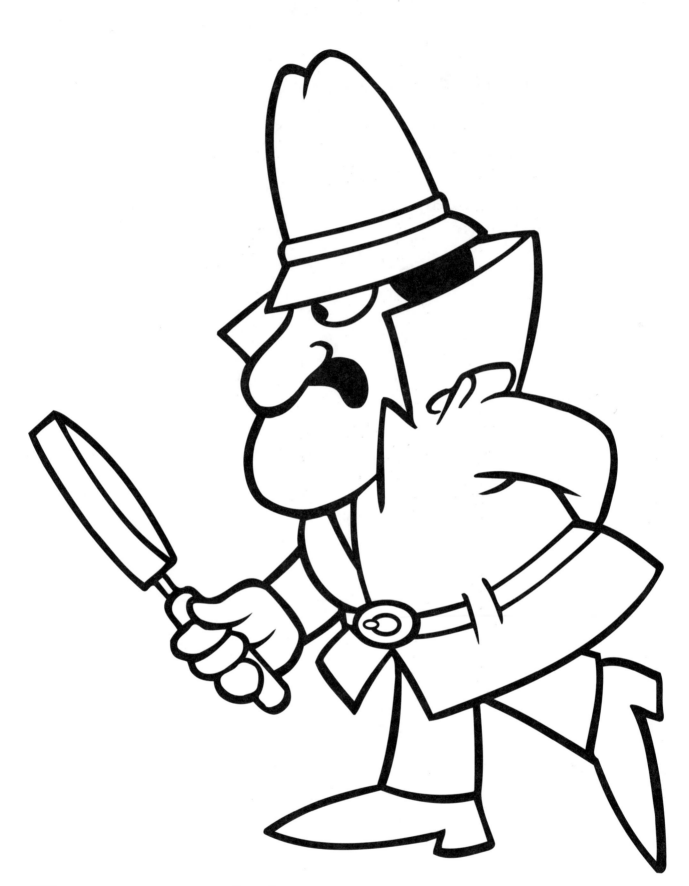

The mystery of what causes type 1 diabetes is now better understood.

Chapter 3
Type 1 Diabetes

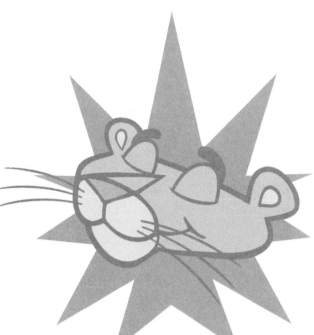

WHAT CAUSES DIABETES?

The cause of type 1 diabetes is believed to be due to three things:

 Genetics: Genes come from both mom and dad and can make someone more likely to get diabetes. Over half of the people that get type 1 diabetes have inherited the gene combination DR3/DR4 (one is from mom and one is from dad).

Self-Allergy (autoimmunity):

- The immune system in the body normally protects it from possible harm.

- An allergy is a reaction by the body's immune system to something it thinks doesn't belong inside the body.

- Self-allergy is when a person's body develops an allergy against one of its own parts. In this case, the allergy is against the islet (eye-let) cells in the pancreas where insulin is made. When the islet cells have been damaged, the immune system makes something called antibodies. These antibodies are present in the blood and are markers of the immune system attacking the pancreas.

Antibodies that may be found in the blood of people with type 1 diabetes are:

- IAA (insulin autoantibody)
- GAD antibody
- ICA512 antibody
- ZnT8 antibody
- Islet cell antibodies (by fluorescent stain)

Sometimes these antibodies are present for many years before the signs of diabetes appear. Half of the people who will someday develop type 1 diabetes already have the antibodies by age five years. Being able to identify antibodies has allowed studies (which have begun in the U.S. and elsewhere) to try to prevent type 1 diabetes (see Chapter 31 on Research).

Virus or Chemical: Having a certain gene makeup may allow a virus or chemical to get to the islet cells (where insulin is made) and cause damage. Once the damage has occurred, the self-allergy likely begins.

TYPE 2 DIABETES

Type 2 (adult-onset) diabetes does not occur as a result of the self-allergy like type 1 diabetes. Therefore, antibodies (found in type 1 diabetes) are not present in the blood. Type 2 diabetes is often associated with being overweight.

Type 2 diabetes has an inherited part (Chapter 4), but the genetics are different from those of type 1 diabetes. As noted in Chapter 4, people with type 2 diabetes may have normal or high insulin levels. The insulin just does not work well. In contrast, people with type 1 diabetes have low or no insulin. The two conditions are both called diabetes. Both result in high sugars, but they are VERY different from each other.

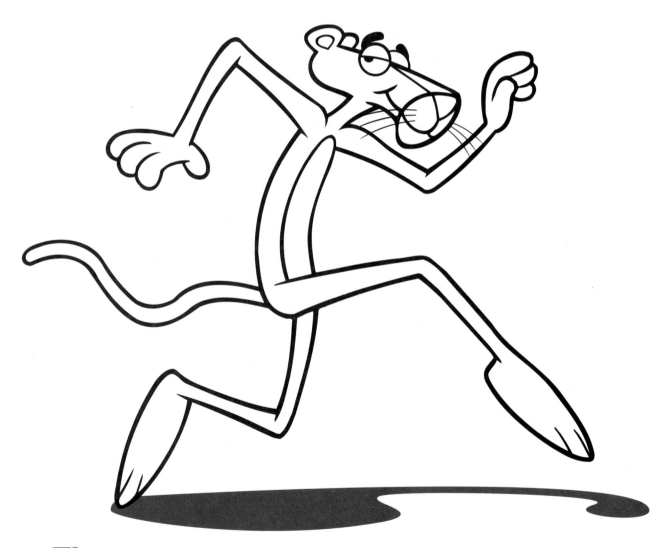

Thirty to sixty minutes of exercise at least five times a week is important for all people.

Chapter 4
Type 2 Diabetes

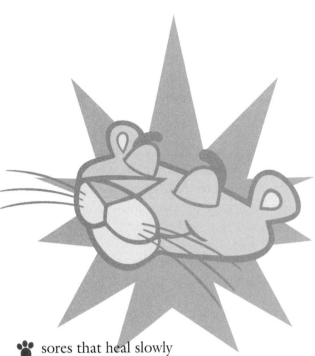

Type 2 diabetes (previously referred to as Adult-onset diabetes or Non-insulin dependent diabetes) is the most common type to occur in adults over age 40 years. It is also becoming more common in youth (particularly in overweight teenagers). It is common in Native-American, African-American and Hispanic youth.

CAUSES

Type 2 diabetes is partly inherited (genetic). It is also linked with being overweight and not getting enough exercise. It is often called a "disease of life-styles." Our ancestors were very active and ate less. We now live in a world of automobile travel, television, computers, video games, and high calorie fast foods.

SYMPTOMS

The symptoms can be the same as with type 1 diabetes (Chapter 2). They may be:

 frequent drinking of liquids

 frequent urination (going to the bathroom)

 infections

 sores that heal slowly

 no energy

 Many people don't have any symptoms. These people are sometimes diagnosed by a high blood sugar that is measured on a routine physical exam or with an elevated hemoglobin A1c (HbA1c) level (see Chapter 14). Others are diagnosed when they have a high blood sugar level on a test called an Oral Glucose Tolerance Test.

TREATMENT: CHANGES IN LIFESTYLE ARE <u>VERY</u> IMPORTANT.

• Eating foods with fewer calories and carbohydrates as well as less fat is needed.

• Getting at least 30 minutes of exercise five to seven days a week is very important.

• Checking blood sugars (like people with type 1 diabetes) is helpful (Chapter 7). The blood sugar values can tell how well the person is doing.

• If at diagnosis a person has ketones, insulin shots are usually needed. The shots may also be needed during times of illness.

- Medications by mouth can be tried if the blood sugar and HbA1c levels return to near normal (Chapter 14). Often by losing weight and exercising, blood sugars do return to near normal.

- The medicines taken by mouth ARE NOT insulin. When taken, these medicines cause the pancreas to make more insulin. They can also make the body more sensitive to its own insulin.

  One of these medicines is called metformin (Glucophage®).

  - This medicine is usually tried first.

  - Rarely, it can cause an upset stomach.

- If a person becomes sick, this medicine should be stopped until they are well. Blood sugars and urine ketones should be checked. Insulin shots may be needed during the illness. Call your doctor or nurse if you are not sure what to do.

- There are other medicines taken by mouth that can be tried if metformin isn't working well.

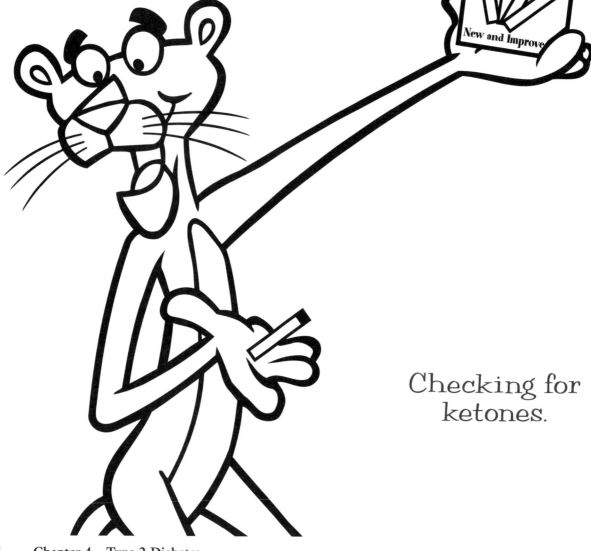

Checking for ketones.

Chapter 5
Checking Ketones

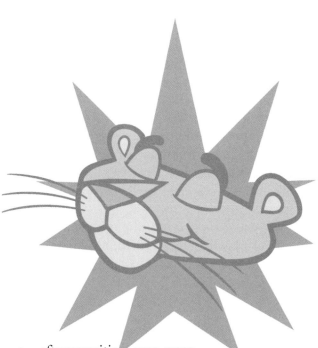

Checking ketones is very easy and very important.

A. FOR A NEWLY DIAGNOSED PERSON:

 The first goal for new patients is to clear their ketones.

Ketones come from fat breakdown. Insulin stops fat breakdown and prevents ketones from being made.

A second goal is to lower blood sugar levels.

Insulin also turns off sugar production from the liver and allows sugar to enter the body's cells.

B. FOR A PERSON WITH KNOWN DIABETES:

When to check for ketones (either in urine or blood):

- during any illness
- with a very high blood sugar (e.g., above 300 mg/dL [>16.7 mmol/L])
- if an insulin shot is missed

- after vomiting even once
- with a blockage of an insulin pump catheter or pump failure

If ketones are present, extra insulin can be given to stop the ketones from being made. (Ketones need to be detected early and extra insulin given or the person may get very sick; see Chapter 15.)

C. HOW TO CHECK FOR KETONES

A method to check for ketones must always be in the home and taken along on trips. Failure to do the ketone check when indicated could result in the person becoming very sick. Ketones can be checked using either urine or a drop of blood. The urine strips are cheaper, although the blood has the advantage of telling how high the ketones are at that moment (as well as other advantages). Some people do the urine ketone check first, and only do the blood ketones if the urine shows moderate or large ketones.

URINE KETONES

The two main strips used are:

1. Ketostix®: available in foil wrapping that allows them to last longer.

This strip is dipped into the urine and is read as negative, trace, small, moderate, large, or extra large after *exactly* 15 seconds.

2. Chemstrip K®: comes in bottles and are not foil wrapped. All non-foil wrapped strips (including non-foil wrapped Ketostix in a bottle) must be thrown out six months after the bottle is opened.

This strip is dipped into the urine and is read as negative, trace, small, moderate, large or extra large after *exactly* 60 seconds.

BLOOD KETONES

Some people prefer to use the Precision Xtra® meter to check blood ketones.

- The purple calibration strip must be placed in the meter first.

- Next, the blood ketone strip is inserted with the three black bars going into the meter.

- Then a drop of blood is placed on the white target area at the end of the strip.

- The result is given in 10 seconds.

Table
Comparison of Blood and Urine Ketone Readings

Blood Ketone	Urine Ketone		Action to take
(mmol/L)	Strip color	Level	
less than 0.6	slight/no color change	negative	normal - no action needed
0.6 to 1.0	light purple	small to moderate	extra insulin & fluids***
1.1 to 3.0	dark purple	moderate to large**	call MD or RN***
greater than 3.0	very dark purple	very large**	go directly to the E.R.

**It is usually advised to call a health care provider for a blood ketone level greater than 1.0 or with urine ketone readings of moderate or large.

***If the blood glucose level is below 150 mg/dL (<8.3 mmol/L), a liquid with sugar (e.g., juice) should be taken so more insulin can be safely given.

Chapter 6
Low Blood Sugar
(Hypoglycemia or Insulin Reaction)

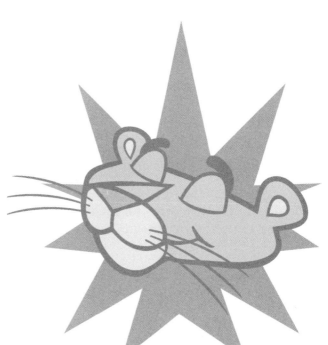

Anyone who has been given insulin can have low blood sugar (hypoglycemia or a "reaction"). Blood sugars below 70 mg/dL (<3.9 mmol/L) are considered low. **A "true low" blood sugar is a value less than 60 mg/dL (3.3 mmol/L).** (Although "blood sugar" is used throughout this chapter, and in many of the chapters, if the person is using a continuous glucose monitor [CGM], it may be the "CGM glucose value").

Main Causes:

 late or missed meals or snacks

 extra exercise (the low may be "delayed" during the night)

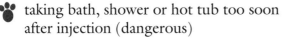 too much insulin/wrong dose

taking bath, shower or hot tub too soon after injection (dangerous)

a previous low blood sugar (for any reason, particularly at bedtime) and failing to do a follow-up blood sugar 15 to 30 minutes later to make sure the value has come up as a result of the treatment

illnesses, especially with vomiting

The signs of a low blood sugar can vary and may include:

hunger

feeling shaky, sweaty and/or weak

confusion

sleepiness (at unusual times)

behavioral/mood changes

double vision

the signs of nighttime lows may be the same, or may include waking up alert, crying, or having bad dreams

Low blood sugar can come on quickly. It must be treated immediately by the person (if able) or by someone who is nearby at the time. If not treated, eventual loss of consciousness or a seizure may occur. Different levels of reactions (mild, moderate, severe) and treatment for each level are shown in the table in this chapter.

With a "mild" low blood sugar (also see Table):

- give sugar (best in liquid form) such as four ounces of juice or sugar pop. Dextrose tablets (usually 3 or 4) also work.

- when possible, a blood sugar should be done.

- it takes 10 to 20 minutes for the blood sugar to rise after treatment.

- re-check the blood sugar after 10 to 20 minutes to make sure the level is above 70 mg/dL (3.9 mmol/L).

- if it is still below this level, the liquid sugar or Dextrose tablets should be given again. Follow the steps above.

- wait another 10 to 15 minutes to repeat the blood sugar level.

- if the blood sugar is above 70 mg/dL (3.9 mmol/L), give solid food. The reason for waiting to give the solid food is that it may soak up the liquid sugar and slow the time for the sugar to get into the blood.

- the person should not return to activity until the blood sugar is above 70 mg/dL (3.9 mmol/L).

- if the low is at bedtime, it is best to repeat the blood sugar, as above, and again during the night to make sure the level stays up.

- if a low blood sugar occurs when it is time for an insulin shot, always treat the low first. Make sure the blood sugar is back up before giving the shot.

With a "moderate" reaction (also see Table):

- put half a tube of Insta-Glucose® or cake gel between the gums and cheeks. Rub the cheeks and stroke the throat to help with swallowing.

If a person has a low blood sugar and can't keep food down or has difficulty getting the value up, low dose glucagon, one unit per year of age up to 15 units, can be given under the skin just like insulin — with an insulin syringe. The dose can be repeated every 20 minutes until the blood sugar is up. Once glucagon is mixed, it usually can continue to be used for about 24 hours before it gels.

With a "severe" reaction (also see Table):

- if a seizure or complete loss of consciousness occurs, it may be necessary to give a shot of glucagon. After mixing, give the following doses under the skin (just like insulin) or into muscle (either works):

  less than 6 years = 0.3 cc (30 units)

  6-16 years = 0.5 cc (50 units)

  greater than 16 years = 1.0 cc (100 units)

Glucagon will make the blood sugar rise, usually in 10 to 20 minutes. Though the result of giving glucagon is the opposite of giving insulin, it is <u>NOT</u> sugar.

Giving glucagon:

 after mixing, it can be given with an insulin syringe just like insulin.

Amount of glucagon to give:

- under 6 years can be given a full 30 unit syringe (0.3 cc).

- 6-16 years can be given a full 50 unit syringe (0.5 cc).

- over 16 years can be given a full 100 unit syringe (1.0 cc).

- if the person does not respond in 10 to 20 minutes the paramedics (911) should be called.

Your doctor or nurse should be called prior to the next insulin shot, as the amount of insulin you give may need to be changed.

Never give a shot and
then get in a shower,
bathtub or hot tub.
The blood coming to the
skin surface may
cause the insulin
to be rapidly
absorbed.
This may result
in a severe
insulin reaction.

Hypoglycemia: Treatment of Low Blood Sugar (B.S.)

Always check blood sugar level!

Low Blood Sugar Category	MILD	MODERATE	SEVERE
Alertness	**ALERT**	**NOT ALERT** **Unable to drink safely (choking risk)** **Needs help from another person**	**UNRESPONSIVE** **Loss of consciousness** **Seizure** **Needs constant adult help (position of safety)** *Give nothing by mouth (extreme choking risk)*
Symptoms	Mood Changes Shaky, Sweaty Hungry Fatigue, Weak Pale	Lack of Focus Headache Confused Disoriented 'Out of Control' (bite, kick) *Can't* Self-treat	Loss of Consciousness Seizure
Actions to take	✔ Check B.S. ✔ Give 2-8 oz sugary fluid (amount age dependent) ✔ Recheck B.S. in 10-15 min. ✔ B.S. > 70 mg/dl (>3.9 mmol/L), repeat sugary fluid and recheck in 10-20 min. ✔ B.S. > 70 mg/dl (>3.9 mmol/L), (give a solid snack)	✔ *Place in position of safety* ✔ Check B.S. ✔ If on insulin pump, may disconnect or suspend until fully recovered from low blood sugar (**awake and alert**). ✔ Give Insta-Glucose or cake decorating gel — put between gums and cheek and rub in. ✔ Look for person to 'wake up' ✔ Recheck B.S. in 10-20 min. ✔ *Once alert* — follow "actions" under 'Mild' column	✔ *Place in position of safety* ✔ Check B.S. ✔ If on insulin pump, disconnect or suspend until fully recovered from low blood sugar (**awake and alert**). ✔ Glucagon — *can be given with an insulin syringe* like insulin: Under 6 years : **30 units (3/10 cc)** 6-16 years: **50 units (1/2 cc)** Over 16 years: **100 units (all of dose or 1 cc)** ✔ If giving 50 or 100 unit doses, may use syringe in box and inject through clothing. ✔ **Check B.S. every 10-15 min. until > 70 mg/dl (>3.9 mmol/L)** ✔ **If no response, may need to call 911** ✔ Check B.S. every hour x 4-5 hours ✔ High risk for more lows x 24 hours *(need to ↑ food intake and ↓ insulin doses)*
Recovery time	10-20 minutes	20-45 minutes	→ Call RN / MD ← and report the episode Effects can last 2-12 hours

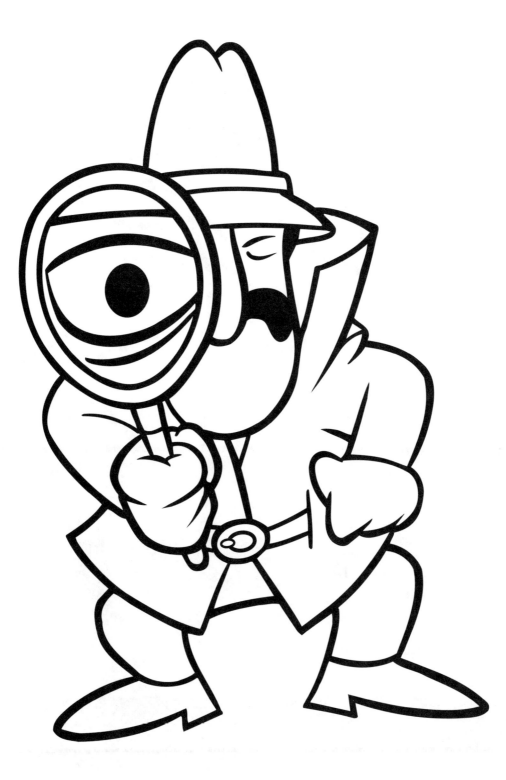

It is important for adults to keep an eye on younger children for signs of low sugar.

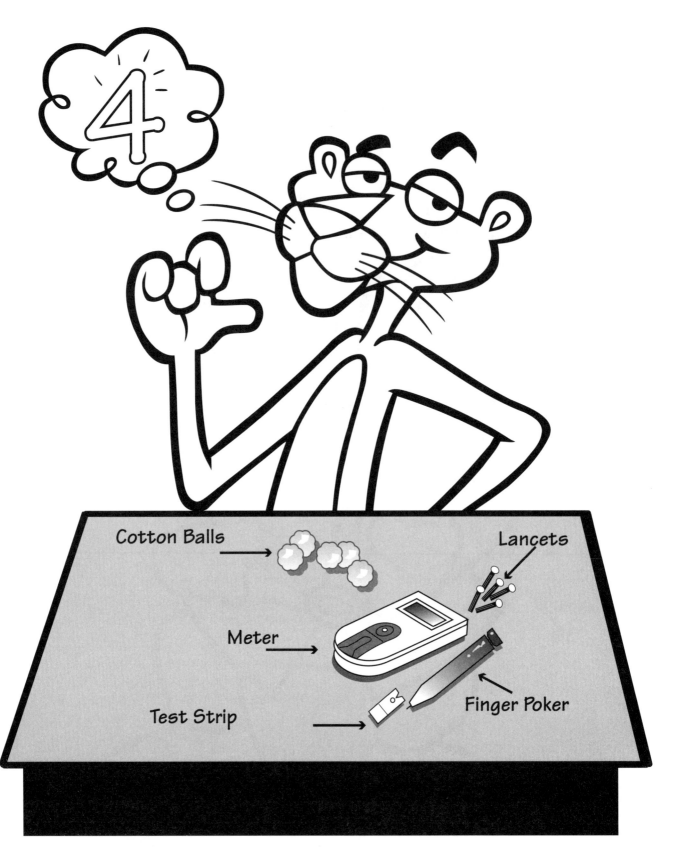

Check your blood sugars four
or more times each day.

Chapter 7

Blood Sugar (Glucose) Monitoring

WHEN?

 four or more times each day (usually before meals and the bedtime snack)

 food should not be eaten within the two hours before a blood sugar determination

 at least once weekly, two hours after each meal

 anytime the symptoms of a low blood sugar are felt

 occasionally during the night

 anytime unusual symptoms occur (e.g., frequent voiding)

GOALS

The target blood sugars are different for each age group and are shown in the table. At least half of the blood sugars at each time of day should be in the desired range for age. The blood sugar ranges refer both to fasting and anytime food has not been eaten for two or more hours.

Table

Blood/CGM Glucose Level in mg/dL (mmol/L) Possible Symptoms

VERY HIGH 400-800 (22.2-44.4)		Stomachache Difficulty Breathing
HIGH 200-400 (11.1-22.2)		Low Energy
GOALS 80-200 (4.5-11.1)	Under 5 years	Fine
70-180 (3.9-10.0)	5-11 years	
70-150 (3.9-8.3)	12 years and up	
LOW below 70 (below 3.9)		Sweating Hunger
"TRUE LOW" below 60 (below 3.3)		Shakiness

NON-DIABETIC NORMAL VALUES FOR CHILDREN*

70-100 (3.9-5.5)	Normal (fasting)*
70-140 (3.9-7.8)	Normal (random)*

*Most values for non-diabetic children are in this range. However, occasional values down to 60 mg/dL (3.3 mmol/L) are still normal.

ALWAYS BRING YOUR METER (and log book) TO YOUR CLINIC VISITS.

DOING THE BLOOD SUGARS

Finger-Pokes: There are now many good devices. Most can be set for different depths. These may help young children or the elderly who do not need a lancet to go as deep.

How to:

 Get poker ready; insert lancet (change daily).

 Wash hands with soap and warm water; dry.

 Poke side or tip (not ball) of chosen finger or of arm (alternate site values; see below).

 To get enough blood, hold hand down (below heart level) and "milk" the finger.

 Put the drop of blood on the blood sugar strip as taught for each meter.

 Hold cotton ball on poke site to stop bleeding.

Meters: We do not recommend one meter over another.

- We do like meters that can store at least the last 100 values.

- The meter must also be able to be downloaded by the family or clinic.

- Strips requiring smaller amounts of blood make it easier for young children.

- Make sure the code in the meter matches the code for the strips (if required).

- **The meter must always be brought to the clinic visit.**

Alternate Site Checking: Some meters now require such a small drop of blood that it can be obtained from the arm or another site. However, if feeling low, the fingertip must be used as circulation is not as good in other sites and the true blood sugar level may be delayed by 10-20 minutes.

Log books: It is important to record results or to download meters at regular intervals.

- Look for patterns of highs and lows.

- If too many lows occur, the results should be sent to the nurse or doctor by fax or email (e.g., more than 2 values per week below 60 mg/dL [3.3 mmol/L]).

- If too many highs occur, the results should be sent to the nurse or doctor by fax or email (e.g., more than 2 values at the same time of day in a week above 300 mg/dL [16.7 mmol/L]).

- We encourage families who send blood sugar results to suggest solutions to their questions, which can be discussed with a doctor or nurse.

- Parents (even of teens) must do or supervise the recording of the values and the sending of the results.

- **Bring the log book to the clinic visit.**

Feelings: It is important not to be upset if highs or lows are found. This can make doing blood sugars a negative experience. Just use the data to adjust the insulin and/or to prevent future highs or lows. We emphasize that sugars are "in target" or "high" or "low" but not "good" or "bad." The only response should be, **"Thank you for doing the blood sugar".**

Continuous Glucose Monitoring (CGM) Diabetes management is gradually moving toward CGM. This involves wearing a sensor for six days each week which will send subcutaneous (not blood) glucose values to a receiver. Some blood sugar checking is still necessary. This is now discussed in Chapter 29.

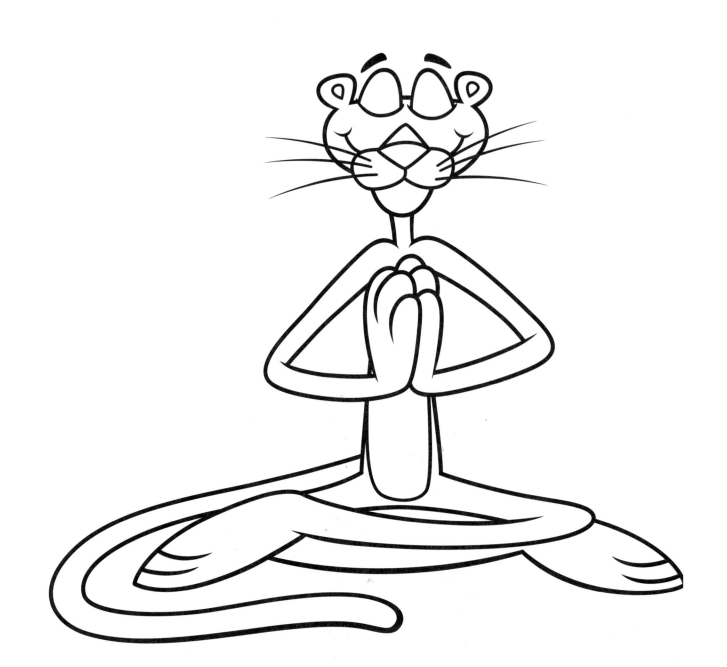

Stay calm, the blood sugar will come down.

Chapter 8
Insulin: Types and Activity

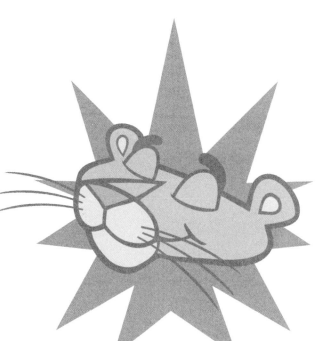

WHY ARE INSULIN SHOTS NEEDED?

 Not enough insulin is made in the pancreas of a person with type 1 diabetes.

 Insulin can't be taken as a pill because it would be destroyed by stomach acid.

 People with type 2 diabetes who have ketones or very high blood sugars also usually take insulin shots, at least in the beginning.

THE THREE TYPES OF INSULIN ARE:

① *"rapid-acting"* (Humalog, NovoLog and Apidra) and Regular

- Humalog, NovoLog and Apidra are more rapid-acting than Regular; they peak earlier and do not last as long as Regular insulin.

- Humalog, NovoLog, Apidra and Regular insulins are clear.

② "intermediate-acting" (NPH)

- NPH insulin is cloudy and must be mixed to get the same dose with each shot.

- The bottles should be turned gently up and down 20 times before drawing the insulin into the syringe.

- NPH insulin peaks 4-6 hours after being given.

③ *"long-acting"* (Lantus® [insulin glargine] and Levemir® [insulin detemir]; see table)

- These are the first true basal (flat-acting, minimal peak) insulins that last approximately 24 hours.

- They are <u>clear</u> insulins (don't confuse with rapid-acting insulins).

- Levemir must be drawn into the syringe alone (cannot be mixed with any other insulin).

- Best given in the bottom (buttocks, seat to make sure the insulin is given into fat) or give into a pinch of fat.

** Insulin must be stored so that it does not freeze or get over 90º F (32° C) because it will spoil.

HOW AND WHEN IS INSULIN USED?

Most people take two or more shots of insulin each day.

RAPID-ACTING INSULIN (HUMALOG, NOVOLOG OR APIDRA):

 Rapid-acting insulins are used to stop the rise of the blood sugar after eating food.

 The rapid-acting insulin can be mixed with NPH insulin to give before breakfast and dinner.

 Most people also take a shot of rapid-acting insulin before lunch and the afternoon snack.

 Rapid-acting insulin should be taken 15-20 minutes before the meal (unless the blood sugar is below 80 mg/dL [4.5 mmol/L]).

 If Regular insulin is being used, the shot is usually taken 30-45 minutes before meals.

 For toddlers the rapid-acting insulin can be given after the meal. Then the dose can be adjusted to fit the amount of food eaten.

 Rapid-acting insulins are also used to "correct" a blood/CGM glucose level that is too high (see Correction Insulin Dose: Chapter 22).

 Regular insulin can be mixed with a rapid-acting insulin to cover high-fat meals (delayed food absorption).

INTERMEDIATE-ACTING INSULIN (NPH):

 NPH insulin has its main effect in 3 to 8 hours and lasts 12 to 15 hours. It is usually taken twice daily in a syringe with a rapid-acting insulin (Figure 1).

- NPH insulin taken at dinner or bedtime has a peak during the night so that low blood sugars are more common compared to when a basal (long-acting) insulin is used.

 People who take three shots per day sometimes take their NPH at bedtime rather than at dinner to help it last through the night.

Figure 1: Example of Two Injections Per Day

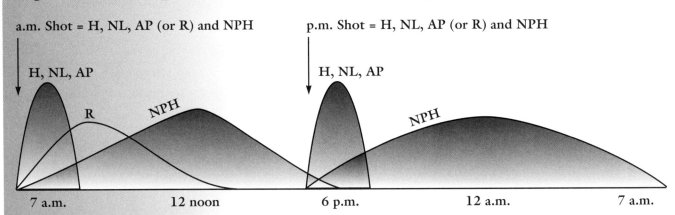

Many people receive two injections per day. NPH and a rapid-acting insulin (or Regular) are given prior to breakfast and dinner. When possible, the insulin should be given 20 minutes prior to the meal.

LONG-ACTING INSULIN (LANTUS OR LEVEMIR):

 When using insulin glargine (Lantus) or insulin detemir (Levemir):

- The dose is usually taken alone without any other insulin in the syringe (ask your doctor). Then Humalog, NovoLog or Apidra are taken 15-20 minutes before each meal (see Figure 2-A).

- It is best to take the insulin in the buttocks (seat) or to give the insulin into a pinch of fat in the stomach (to make sure the insulin is going into the fat).

- The action is very flat and the chance for a low blood sugar is reduced (particularly during the night when the basal insulin is taken in the morning).

- It works as a basal insulin, which prevents the liver from producing sugar and ketones and releasing them into the blood.

- NPH (an intermediate-acting insulin) is sometimes taken in the morning, particularly if a noon shot cannot be taken. It can be given in the same syringe with the rapid-acting insulin. See example in Figure 2-B.

- The dose is judged on the basis of the morning blood sugar no matter when the Lantus or Levemir shot is taken (a.m., lunch, dinner or bedtime; all times work - though one consistent time must be chosen). If the blood sugar is consistently above the desired range at breakfast (Chapter 7), the dose is increased. If below the lower level, the dose is decreased.

Figure 2: Use of Lantus or Levemir Insulin

Two of the most common methods of using Lantus or Levemir insulin:

Figure 2-A. In the first example, Lantus or Levemir is used as the basal insulin (given in the a.m., or at dinner or at bedtime) and a rapid-acting insulin is taken 15-20 minutes prior to meals and snacks.

Figure 2-B. In this second example, NPH and a rapid-acting insulin are taken in one syringe 15-20 minutes prior to breakfast. A rapid-acting insulin is taken alone 15-20 minutes prior to dinner. Lantus or Levemir (alone in the syringe) is taken consistently either in the a.m., at dinner, or at bedtime.

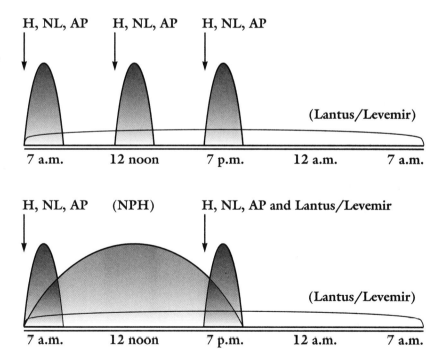

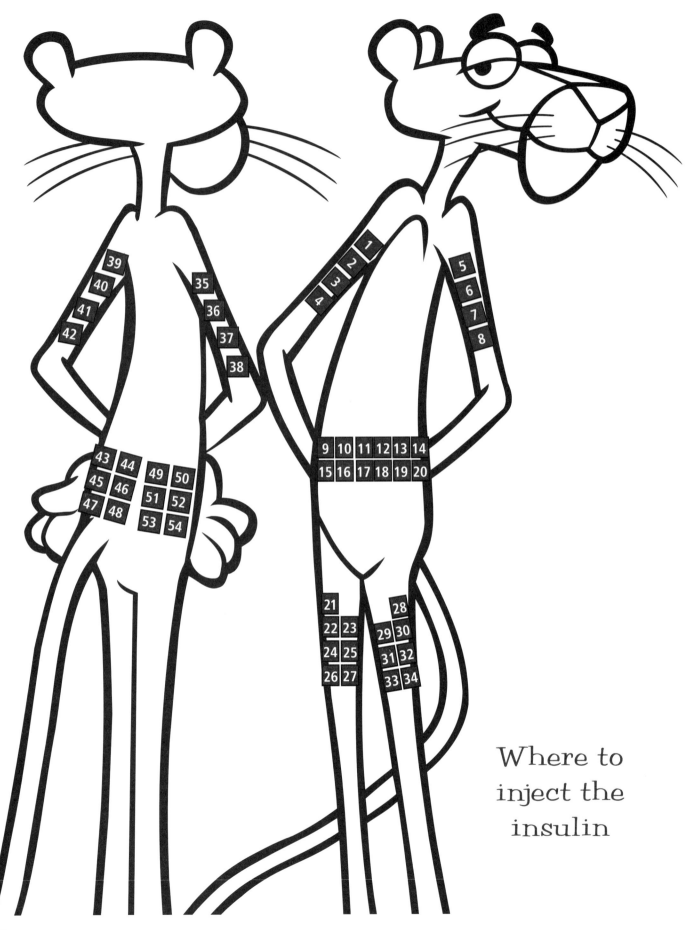

Where to
inject the
insulin

Chapter 9

Drawing Up and Giving Insulin

The nurse-educator will teach the best way to draw up and give the insulin. Both are described below and in Figures 1 and 2.

DRAWING UP INSULIN

A. <u>Get everything you will need:</u>

- a bottle of each insulin you will use

- syringe

- alcohol wipe for tops of bottles

- log book with current blood sugar results and insulin dose: please record each blood sugar result and insulin dose in log book

B. <u>What to do (example of drawing up two insulins into a syringe):</u>

- Know how much of each insulin you need to give (based on "thinking" scales if appropriate – see Chapter 22 in "*Understanding Diabetes*").

- Wipe off the tops of insulin bottles with alcohol swab.

- Inject air into the intermediate-acting (cloudy) insulin bottle with the bottle sitting upright on the table and remove the needle.*

- Inject air in the clear (rapid-acting) insulin bottle and leave the needle in the bottle.*

- Turn the rapid-acting bottle with the needle in it upside down and get rid of any air bubbles. (See this chapter in "*Understanding Diabetes*" for specific steps that can be used to get rid of air bubbles.) Draw up the clear rapid-acting insulin you need and remove the needle from the bottle.

- Mix the cloudy (NPH) insulin by gently turning the bottle up and down 20 times; this mixes the insulin so that it will have a consistent strength.

- Turn the bottle upside down and put the needle into the bottle. Draw up the cloudy insulin into the syringe. *Make sure not to push any rapid-acting insulin already in the syringe back into this bottle.*

- If the insulin bottles have been in the refrigerator, you can warm up the insulin once it is mixed in the syringe by holding the syringe in the closed palm of your hand for a minute. It will be less likely to sting if the insulin is at room temperature.

*An option now used by some people is to not put air into the insulin bottles, but to just "vent" the bottles once a week to remove any vacuum. This is done by removing the plunger from the syringe and inserting the needle into the upright insulin bottle. Air will be sucked in through the needle removing the vacuum from the bottle. (The vacuum may otherwise pull insulin from the syringe into the insulin bottle. This is most important if two insulins are being mixed in the same syringe.)

Figure 1

GIVING THE INSULIN

 Choose the area of the body where you are going to give the shot. Use two or more areas and use different sites within the area.

 Make sure the area where you will be giving the shot is clean.

Relax the chosen area.

Pull up the skin with the finger and thumb (even with short needles).

Touch the needle to the skin and "punch" it through the skin.

Short Needle
- a 90° angle for the 5/16 inch (short) or the BD Ultra-Fine Nano needle: (these hurt less and are not as likely to go into muscle)
  (a 90° angle looks like this: ___↓___)

Long Needle
- use a 45° angle for the 5/8 inch needle (only)
  (a 45° angle looks like this: ___↘___)

Push in the insulin slowly and steadily; wait 10 seconds to let the insulin spread out.

Let go of the skin pulled up.

Put a finger or dry cotton over the needle as it is pulled out; gently rub a few times to close the hole where the needle was inserted; press your finger or the cotton down on the area where you gave the shot if bruising or bleeding happens.

Look to see if a drop of insulin comes back through the hole the needle made ("leak-back"); make a note in your log book if this happens.

The nurse will teach the right way to give shots so that a drop of insulin does not leak-back. A drop can contain as much as five units of insulin.

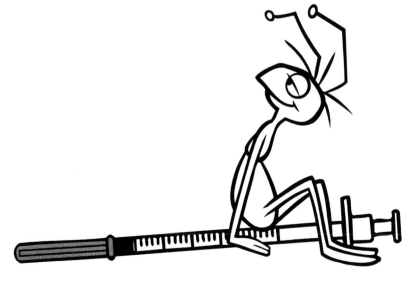

Figure 2
Injecting the Insulin

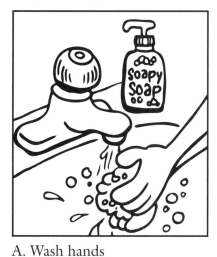

A. Wash hands

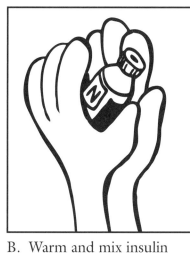

B. Warm and mix insulin

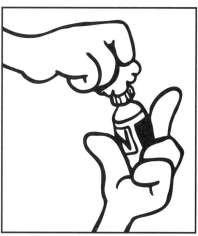

C. Wipe top of insulin bottle with alcohol

D. Inject air=insulin dose in units

Pull out dose of insulin

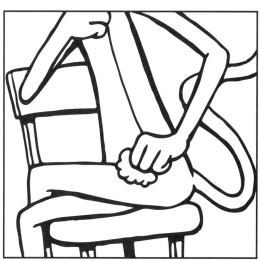

E. Make sure injection site is clean

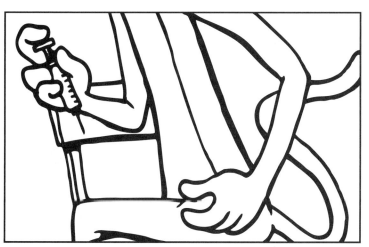

F. Pinch up skin and fat tissue.

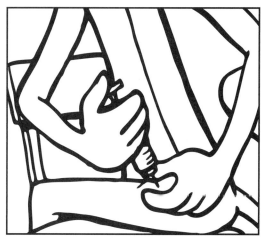

G. Inject insulin.

INSULIN PENS

 Insulin pens have become more popular in recent years.

 They give accurate insulin dosages, but must prime before each injection.

 The injection should be slow and followed by a 10 second wait to remove the needle.

 They are convenient to use at school and when away from home.

WHEN TO INJECT THE INSULIN

When possible, the rapid-acting insulin should be given 15 to 20 minutes prior to the meal (young children who do not eat consistently are the exception). Blood/CGM glucose levels from food peak in 60 minutes whereas the Humalog, Novolog or Apidra peak in 90 minutes (see Figure 3).

CHILDREN AND INSULIN SHOTS

 A young child can help with choosing where the shot will be given (although sites must be rotated) and by holding still.

 Children usually begin to give some of their own shots around age 10.

 It is important that both mom and dad share in giving shots.

 Some age-related issues (see Chapter 18) are:

Toddlers:

• This age group can sometimes be frightened when having to get shots.

• Some toddlers are helped by the Insuflon® or the I-Port (see this chapter in "*Understanding Diabetes*").

Figure 3
(Reproduced with permission of Diabetes Technology and Therapeutics 12:173, 2010)

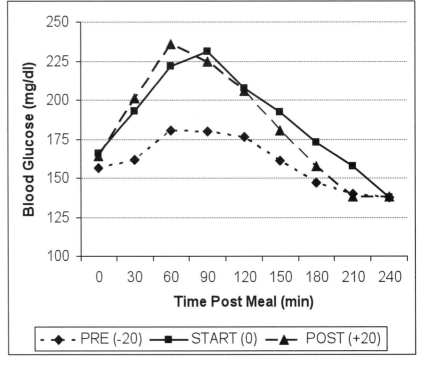

Blood sugar levels when insulin was given 20 minutes prior to a meal ("PRE"), at the beginning of the meal ("START"), or after the meal ("POST"). The ADA goal for blood sugars at any time after a meal is to not exceed 180 mg/dL (10 mmol/L).

- Keep the area where the shot will be given as still as possible. Try to get the child's attention on something else (e.g., television, blowing bubbles, looking at a book, etc.). This will help the child to relax.

- The buttocks are often used first, and later the legs and arms and tummy.

- With the child's permission, the Lantus or Levemir insulin can be given when the child is asleep.

- The parent must remember when giving their child a shot they are giving them health.

School age:

- The child may help in choosing the area on their body to give the shot.

- Change where the shots are given. Use two or more areas and use different sites within the area.

Teens:

- Many teens give their own shots and do not want help.

- It is still important to give the shots in a place (e.g., the kitchen) where parents can actually see the shot given.

- Parents can stay involved by helping to get the supplies out, and helping to keep records by writing down the blood sugars and insulin doses each day in the log book or by emailing CGM downloads.

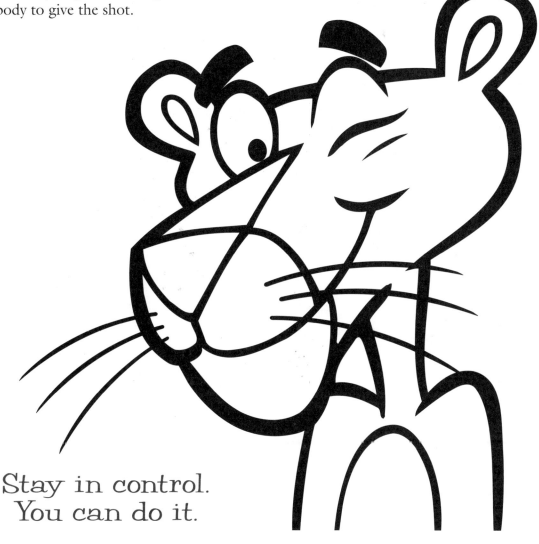

Stay in control.
You can do it.

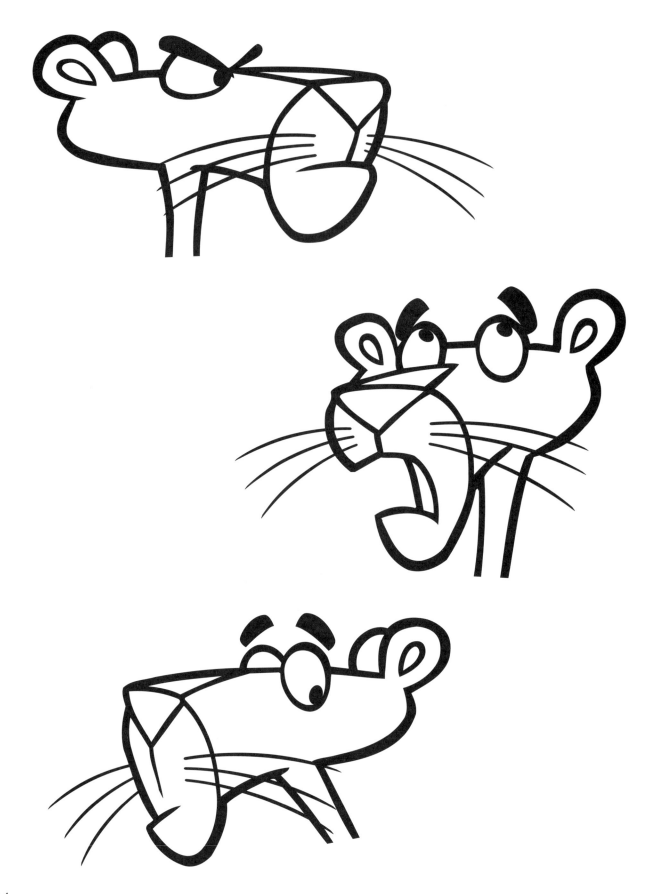

Chapter 10
Feelings and Diabetes

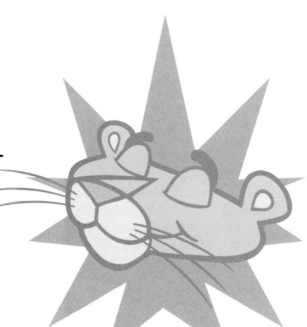

You and your child will have many feelings when you find out about the diabetes. Having these feelings is very normal. It is important for families to share and talk about these feelings.

The most common feelings are:

- **shock**
- **grief**
- **denial**
- **sadness**
- **anger**
- **fear/anxiety**
- **guilt**
- **adapting: as time passes, everyone will not feel so overwhelmed**

Each of these feelings is discussed in detail in the larger book, *"Understanding Diabetes"* (order form in back).

We ask **EVERY** newly diagnosed family to meet with a counselor to discuss feelings. It is important for all family members to share how they feel. All family members need to work toward feeling positive about how diabetes will fit into their family life.

As time passes, the family will find they are better able to deal with the shots, blood sugar checks, food plan and other daily tasks. More talking within the family and with their health care givers can help reduce the stress.

Fitting the diabetes into as normal a lifestyle as possible becomes the major goal.

Adjustment continues to improve after the first few weeks, the first few months and even after the first few years.

The Healthy Eating Pyramid

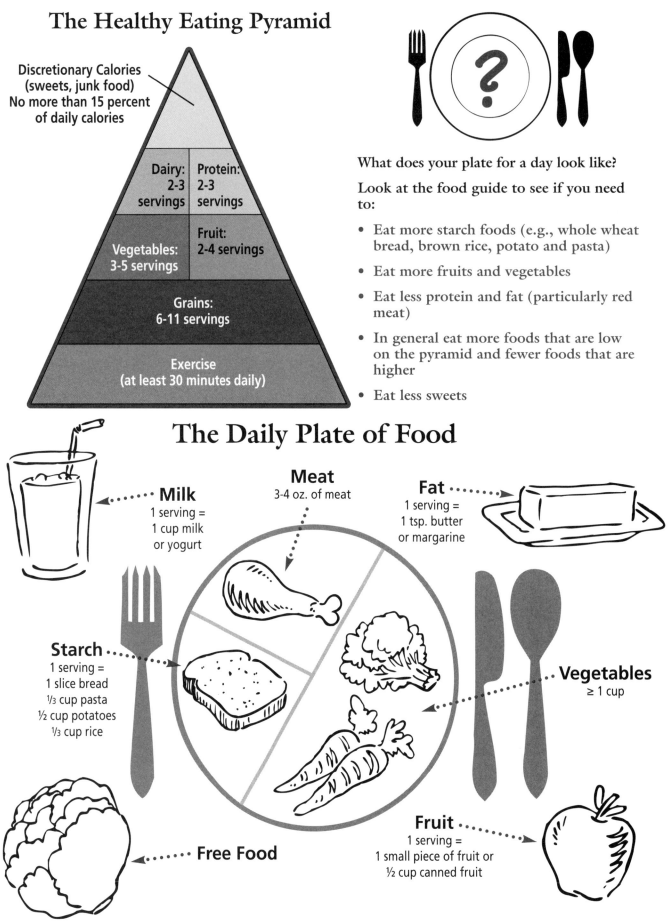

Discretionary Calories (sweets, junk food) No more than 15 percent of daily calories

Dairy: 2-3 servings

Protein: 2-3 servings

Fruit: 2-4 servings

Vegetables: 3-5 servings

Grains: 6-11 servings

Exercise (at least 30 minutes daily)

What does your plate for a day look like?

Look at the food guide to see if you need to:

- Eat more starch foods (e.g., whole wheat bread, brown rice, potato and pasta)
- Eat more fruits and vegetables
- Eat less protein and fat (particularly red meat)
- In general eat more foods that are low on the pyramid and fewer foods that are higher
- Eat less sweets

The Daily Plate of Food

Milk
1 serving =
1 cup milk
or yogurt

Meat
3-4 oz. of meat

Fat
1 serving =
1 tsp. butter
or margarine

Starch
1 serving =
1 slice bread
⅓ cup pasta
½ cup potatoes
⅓ cup rice

Vegetables
≥ 1 cup

Free Food

Fruit
1 serving =
1 small piece of fruit or
½ cup canned fruit

Chapter 11
Normal Nutrition

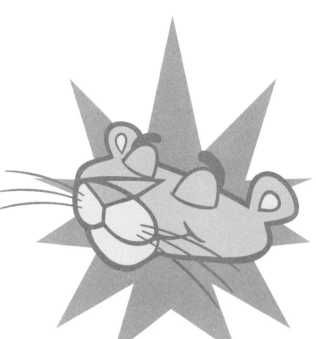

Some knowledge of normal nutrition helps when working with the dietitian on a diabetes food plan.

The foods we eat are divided into:

- **proteins - 4 calories per gram eaten**
- **carbohydrates (includes all sugars: 4 calories per gram eaten)**
- **fats - 9 calories per gram eaten**
- **vitamins and minerals**
- **water**
- **fiber**

All of these are important for our bodies and are discussed in more detail in *"Understanding Diabetes"*. We emphasize with patients and families that the ideal diet for someone with diabetes is really just a healthy diet from which all people would benefit.

Some people with type 2 diabetes can be treated with diet and exercise alone. This is not true for type 1 diabetes. In recent years people with type 1 diabetes have also tended to be heavier. This results in more insulin resistance. Reduction of high fat foods and portion control (along with exercise) are important for everyone.

Insulin has its main effect on sugars and a goal of treatment is matching insulin to carbohydrate intake.

It is important to think about the following:

- **WHEN** carbohydrate is eaten. (Do not constantly snack between meals, or else blood/CGM glucose levels will be high.)

- **HOW MUCH** carbohydrate is eaten. (A can of sugar-sweetened pop has 10 teaspoons of sugar and is unhealthy for anyone.)

- **WITH WHAT** the carbohydrate is eaten. (Other foods, such as fat, slow the sugar absorption.)

- **IF INSULIN IS ACTING** at the same time the sugar is eaten, which allows the sugar to pass into cells for energy rather than out into the urine (see Chapter 2).

Other thoughts discussed in Chapter 11 of *"Understanding Diabetes"* are:

- Working with the dietitian helps families keep up-to-date on new dietary ideas.

- Learning to read nutrition labels on foods at the store is very important.

- Having normal levels of blood fats (e.g., total cholesterol and LDL cholesterol) is important for all people. These levels can be checked once yearly at a clinic visit.

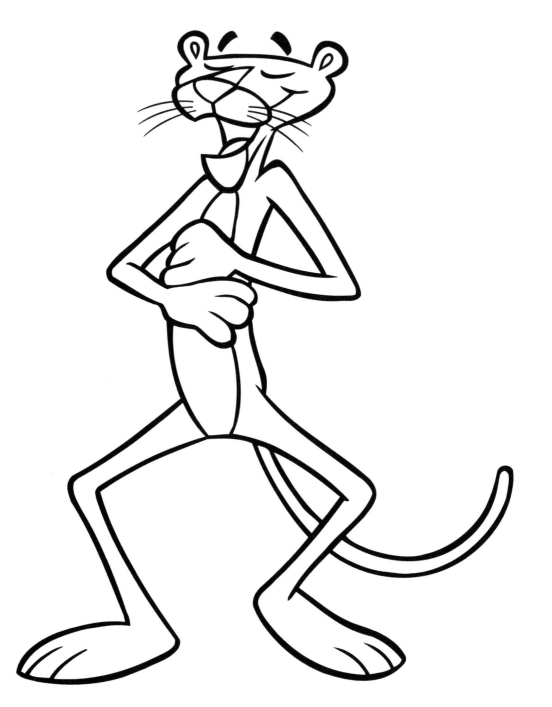

Eating nutritious foods
will help all family members.

Chapter 12
Food Management and Diabetes

A food plan is important for people with either type 1 or type 2 diabetes. Every family must work out a plan with their dietitian that fits their family.

Type 1 diabetes <u>cannot</u> be treated with diet alone.

All people with diabetes should focus on a healthy, balanced diet (see Chapter 12 in *"Understanding Diabetes"*).

People with type 2 diabetes:

 can sometimes be treated with diet and exercise alone

 need to:

- eat foods with fewer calories and smaller portion sizes to lose weight

- avoid concentrated sweets (such as pop containing sugar)

- reduce fat content in their diet

- avoid unhealthy choices at fast food restaurants (burger, fries, pizza)

The two types of food plans that our clinic uses the most are:

① Constant carbohydrate: A family often starts with this plan.

- This plan involves eating about the same amount of carbs for each meal and for each snack from day to day.

- Insulin doses are changed based on the blood/CGM glucose levels, exercise, and other factors such as illness, stress, menses, etc. ("thinking scale").

② Carbohydrate ("carb") counting: Families often move to this plan at a later date.

- This plan involves counting the grams of carbohydrate (carbs) in food to be eaten. An amount of rapid-acting insulin is given that matches the number of grams (g) of carbohydrate (I/C ratio = insulin to carb ratio).

- The healthcare team and family choose an insulin-to-carb ratio (I/C ratio).

- The dietitian may want a three-day diet record to be done first (see Chapter 11 in "Understanding Diabetes").

- The ratio used when starting this plan depends on the patient. An example is one unit of insulin for each 15g of carbohydrate (I/C ratio of 1 to 15).

- Blood/CGM glucose levels are then evaluated 2 to 4 hours after meals to see if the I/C ratio is correct.

  If the blood/CGM glucose level is high (e.g., over 180 mg/dL or 10.0 mmol/L), the ratio could be changed to one unit of insulin for 10g of carbs (I/C ratio of 1 to 10).

  If the blood/CGM glucose level is low (e.g., less than 60 mg/dL or 3.3 mmol/L), the ratio could be changed to one unit of insulin for 20g of carbs (I/C ratio of 1 to 20).

- Gradually the correct ratios for each meal are found. The I/C ratio may vary between meals.

- A blood/CGM glucose level is evaluated and an insulin dose "correction factor" (see Chapter 22) is usually added to the I/C ratio dose. This will be the total dose of insulin to be given 15 to 20 minutes before the meal or snack.

- If blood/CGM glucose levels are above the desired upper level one or two hours after meals (and the pre-meal blood/CGM glucose level is above 90 mg/dL [5.0 mmol/L]), it may be helpful to give the pre-meal rapid-acting insulin 15 to 20 minutes before meals. This is because blood/CGM glucose levels peak in 60 minutes after a meal, whereas Humalog/NovoLog/Apidra insulins do not peak until 90 minutes after injection.

Several tables of the carb contents of foods and more details about carb counting are found in Chapter 12 of *"Understanding Diabetes"*.

Some beginning rules of food management, some of which relate more to a constant carb food plan, are:

- eat a well-balanced diet

- keep the diet similar from day to day

- eat meals and snacks at the same time each day

- watch the portion size of foods to be eaten

- snacks may be needed to prevent insulin reactions, especially with exercise (see suggested snacks in Chapter 12 of *"Understanding Diabetes"*)

- carefully watch how much carbohydrate is eaten

- avoid over-treating low blood sugars

- eat foods with less cholesterol and saturated fats; reduce total fat intake

- keep appropriate growth

- watch weight for height; avoid becoming overweight

- increase the amount of fiber eaten

- eat fewer foods that are high in salt (sodium)

- avoid eating too much protein

- complete 2010 dietary guidelines are available at www.dietaryguidelines.gov

A study known as the **DCCT*** found six dietary factors that made sugar control better:

 following some sort of a meal plan

 not eating extra snacks

 not over-treating low blood sugars (hypoglycemia)

 prompt treatment of high blood sugars when found

 adjusting insulin levels for meals

consistency of bedtime snacks

As shown in the diagram in Chapter 14, food and exercise are two of the four major influences on sugar control. Both are important if excess weight is present or is to be avoided.

*DCCT: Diabetes Control and Complications Trial (see Chapter 14)

If you have had heavy exercise, or if the blood/CGM glucose level sugar is below 130 mg/dL (7.3 mmol/L) or if a peak (NPH) insulin is taken at night then make sure you eat a bedtime snack that has solid protein, fat and carbohydrate. Otherwise, if basal insulins are used, and the blood/CGM glucose level is above 130 mg/dL (>7.3 mmol/L) a bedtime snack may not be required (as they can lead to unhealthy weight gain).

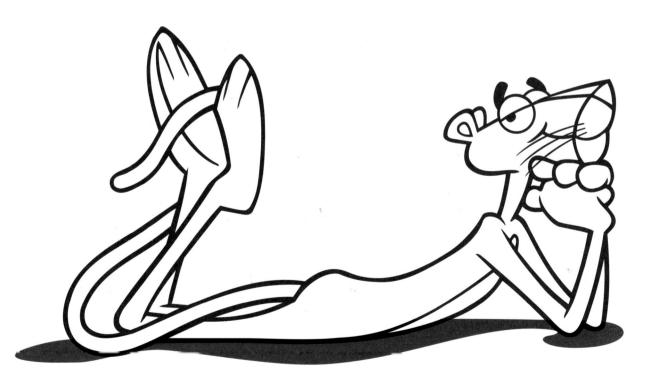

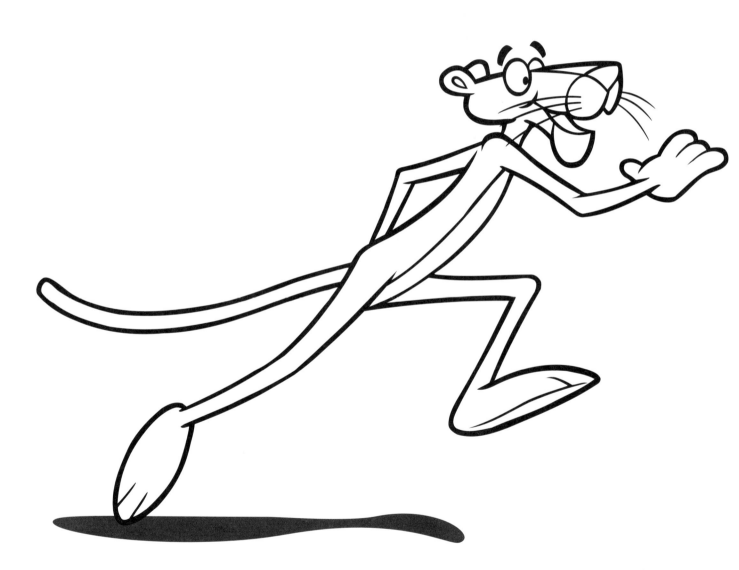

Getting plenty of exercise is important
for everyone.

Chapter 13
Exercise and Diabetes

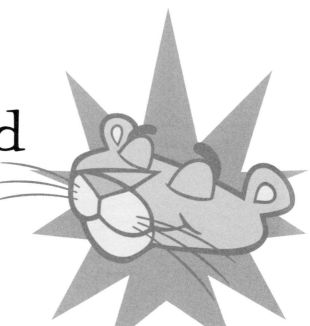

Regular exercise is important for everyone. It may be even more important for people with diabetes. Many former and present professional athletes have diabetes (see *"Understanding Diabetes,"* Chapter 13).

For people with type 2 diabetes, regular exercise and eating less food are two of the most important parts of treating the diabetes (see Chapter 4).

Blood Sugars With and Without One Hour of Exercise

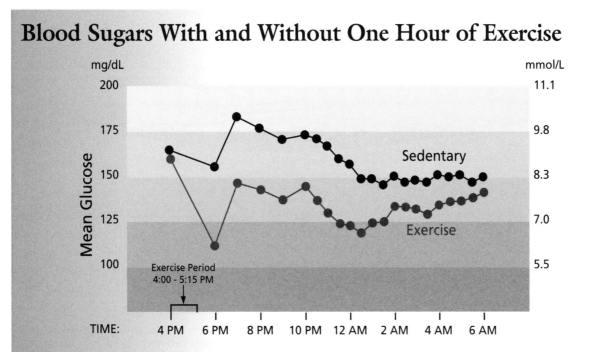

This Figure presents blood glucose (sugar) levels for the same 50 children on a sedentary day (black circles) and an exercise day (red circles). The one hour of exercise at 4 p.m. resulted in lower blood sugar levels for the next 14 hours (through the night). Insulin doses and food intake were identical for the two days.

(Data complements of the DirecNet Study Group: J Pediatr 147,528, 2005)

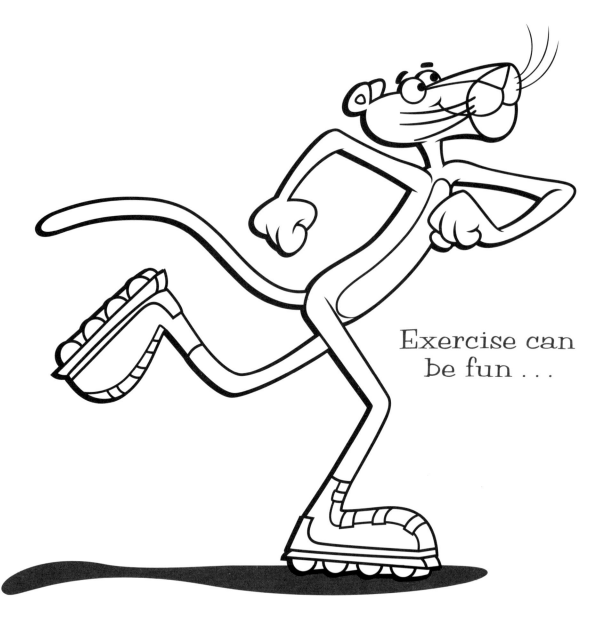

Exercise can
be fun . . .

EXERCISE:

- is one of the "big four," which, along with insulin or oral medicines, food and stress affects blood/CGM glucose levels (see figure in Chapter 14).

- may lower or raise (due to adrenaline output) the blood/CGM glucose levels. Over-all, exercise helps to keep the blood/CGM glucose values in a good range. It does this in part by making us more sensitive to insulin.

- is a primary part of treating type 2 diabetes

- is essential for weight control

- should be done daily for at least 30 to 60 minutes by people with type 1 or type 2 diabetes

- can cause **low blood/CGM glucose values** (Chapter 6) so it is important to plan ahead

The following may help:

- Extra snacks or less insulin may be needed.

- Aiming for a higher blood/CGM glucose level before exercise (e.g., 180 mg/dL [10.0 mmol/L]).

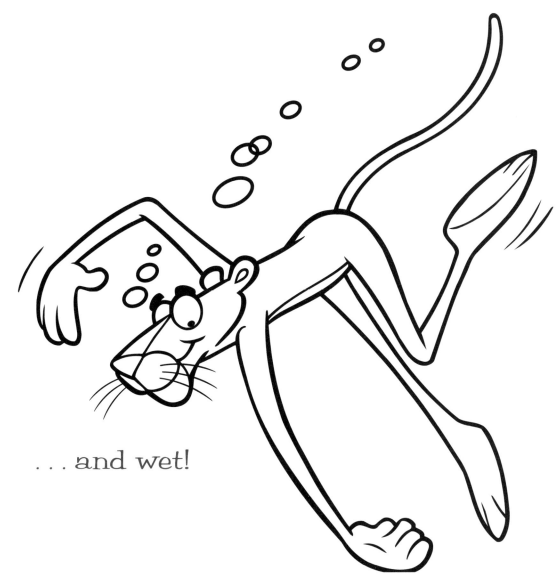

... and wet!

- Thinking ahead to prevent low blood sugars during or up to 12 hours after the exercise ("delayed hypoglycemia").

  ~ The evening insulin dose may need to be reduced.

  ~ Adding an extra 15 or 30 grams of carbohydrate at bedtime if afternoon or evening exercise has been strenuous.

  ~ Making sure the bedtime blood/CGM glucose value is above 130 mg/dL (7.3 mmol/L).

- Use of drinks such as Gatorade® during hard exercise.

- Doing extra blood/CGM glucose levels can be very helpful.

- Drinking extra water during exercise prevents dehydration.

- Eventually, use of an insulin pump makes insulin adjustments easier to prevent exercise-related hypoglycemia.

- Some insulin-pump users who disconnect from their pump during exercise can benefit by giving part of their basal insulin as Lantus or Levemir and part via the pump.

- Regular exercise may also be important for people with diabetes in helping to keep normal foot circulation in later years.

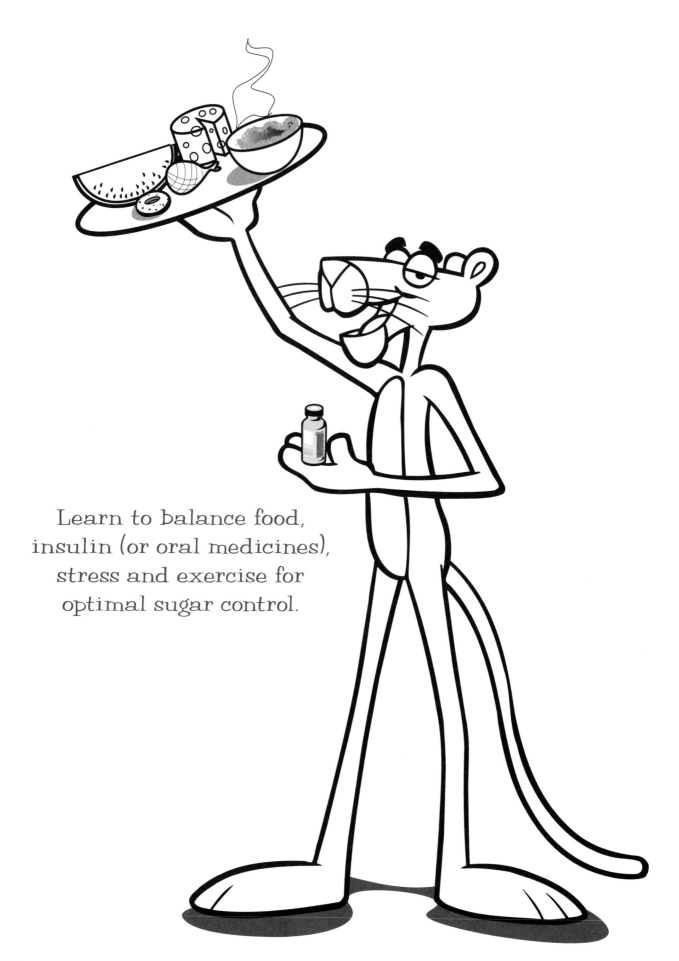

Learn to balance food,
insulin (or oral medicines),
stress and exercise for
optimal sugar control.

Chapter 14

Monitoring Blood/CGM Glucose and HbA1c Levels

A goal for the management of diabetes is to have blood/CGM glucose levels as close to the levels of someone without diabetes as is safely possible.

SUGAR CONTROL:

- is measured day to day by checking blood sugar levels on a meter or, more recently, by a continuous glucose monitor (CGM).

- is monitored for the longer term by a very important measurement called the hemoglobin A1c (**HbA1c or A1c**).

The HbA1c value:

- can be thought of as the **"forest"** and the blood/CGM glucose values as the **"trees"**

- tells how often the sugars have been high for every second of the day for the past 90 days

- should be done every three months

- should be in the desired range (see table) for a person to be in "optimal sugar control"

WHY IS SUGAR CONTROL IMPORTANT?

Optimal Sugar Control:

 helps people feel better.

 can lessen the risk for the eye, kidney, nerve and heart problems from diabetes. This was proven by The **DCCT** (**D**iabetes **C**ontrol and **C**omplications **T**rial).

 helps to lower blood fats (cholesterol and triglyceride levels; see Chapter 11).

 may include reduction of the wide "swings" in blood/CGM glucose levels.

helps children grow to their full adult height.

Table 1
ADA*-Recommended HbA1c and Blood Glucose Values
(ADA: 2010*)

	(Hemoglobin A1c) HbA1c Values	Blood Glucose : mg/dL (mmol/L) Fasting/Before Meals	Bedtime/Overnight
Normal (Non-diabetic):	≤ 5.9%	70-100** (3.9-5.5)	70-120** (3.9-6.7)
Desired ranges for someone with diabetes:			
below six years	7.5-8.5%	100-180 (5.5-10.0)	110-200 (6.1-11.1)
6-12 years	< 8.0%	90-180 (5.0-10.0)	100-180 (5.5-10.0)
13-19 years	< 7.5%	90-130 (5.0-7.3)	90-150 (5.0-8.3)
> 19 years	< 7.0%	90-130 (5.0-7.3)	— —

*ADA *"Diabetes Care"* 33 (Suppl 1, S4), 2010
**Data from JDRF CGM Study Group, Diabetes Care 33, 1297, 2010

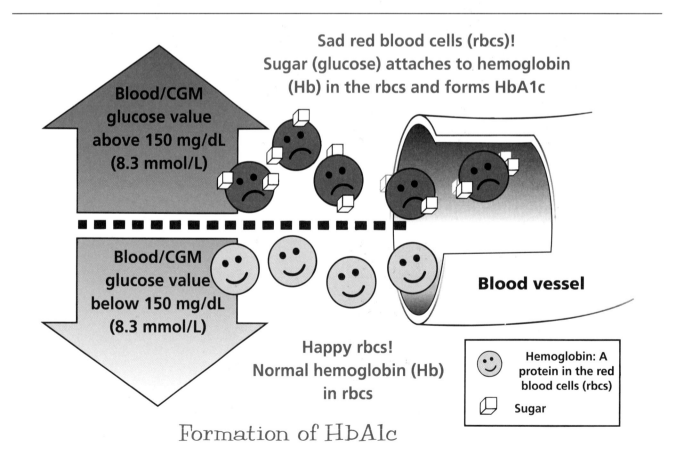

Formation of HbA1c

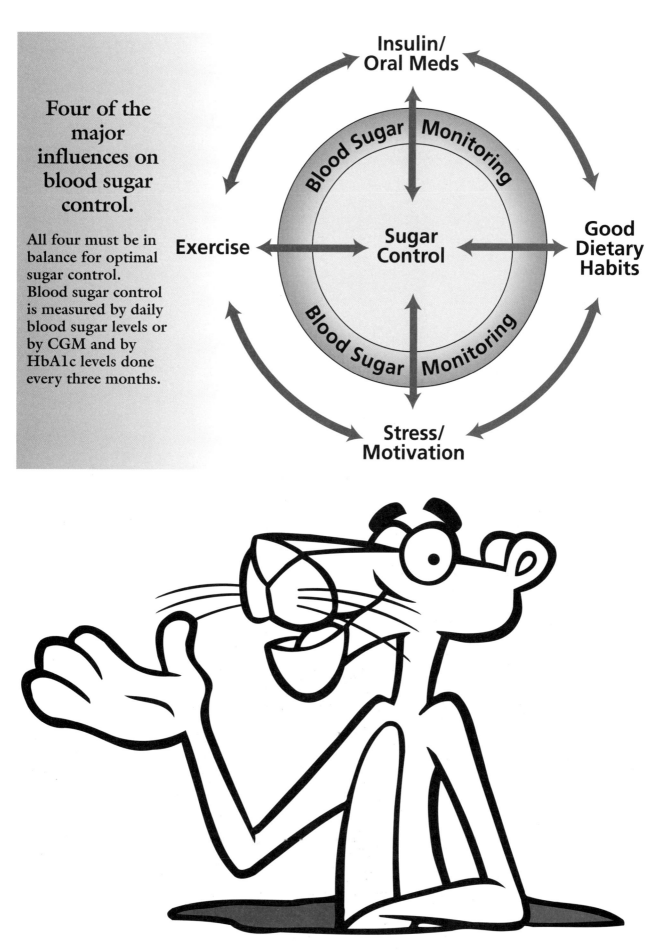

Four of the major influences on blood sugar control.

All four must be in balance for optimal sugar control. Blood sugar control is measured by daily blood sugar levels or by CGM and by HbA1c levels done every three months.

Insulin/
Oral Meds

Blood Sugar Monitoring

Exercise

Sugar
Control

Good
Dietary
Habits

Blood Sugar Monitoring

Stress/
Motivation

Table
The Two Emergencies of Diabetes

	Low Blood Sugar (Chapter 6) (Hypoglycemia or Insulin Reaction)	Ketoacidosis (Chapter 15) (Acidosis or DKA)
Due to:	Low blood sugar	Presence of ketones
Time of onset:	Fast – within minutes	Slow – in hours or days
Causes:	Too little food Too much insulin Too much exercise without food Missing or being late for meals/snacks Excitement in young children	Too little insulin Not giving insulin Infections/Illness Traumatic body stress Pump insertions malfunctioning
Blood sugar:	Low (below 60 mg/dL or 3.3 mmol/L)	Usually high (over 240 mg/dL or 13.3 mmol/L)
Ketones:	Usually none in the urine or blood	Usually moderate/large in the urine or blood ketones over 0.6 mmol/L.
Mild:	**SYMPTOMS** Hunger, shaky, sweaty, nervous **TREATMENT** Give juice or milk. Wait 10 minutes and then give solid food.	**SYMPTOMS** Thirst, frequent urination, sweet breath, small or moderate urine ketones or blood ketones less than 1.0 mmol/L. **TREATMENT** Give lots of fluids and Humalog/NovoLog/Apidra **or** Regular insulin every two or three hours.
Moderate:	Give instant glucose or a fast-acting sugar, juice or sugar pop (4 oz). After 10 minutes, give solid food.	Dry mouth, nausea, stomach cramps, vomiting, moderate or large urine ketones or blood ketones between 1.0 and 3.0 mmol/L. Continued contact with healthcare provider. Give lots of fluids. Give Humalog/NovoLog/Apidra or Regular insulin every two or three hours. Give Zofran (a tablet) or Phenergan medication (suppository or topical cream) if vomiting occurs.
Severe:	Loss of consciousness or seizures. Occurs after being low for a prolonged time. Give glucagon into muscle or fat. Check blood sugar. If no response, call paramedic (911) or go to E.R.	Labored deep breathing, extreme weakness, confusion and eventually unconsciousness (coma): large urine ketones or blood ketones above 3.0 mmol/L. *Go to the emergency room.* May need intravenous fluids and insulin.

Chapter 15
Ketones and Acidosis

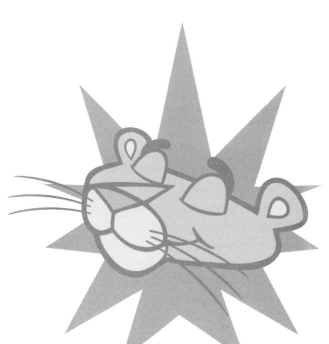

This is the second emergency (the other being low blood sugar) and is more common in type 1 than type 2 diabetes (but can occur in type 2 diabetes).

WHAT LEADS TO DKA?

DKA occurs when *ketones* build up in the body because there isn't enough insulin. DKA is avoidable in a person with known diabetes.

Ketones are:

- made by the body from breaking down fat when sugar cannot be used for energy (not enough insulin in the body)

- an acid that forms when the body uses fat for the energy it needs

HOW DOES IT START?

- The body makes ketones when there isn't enough insulin. Ketones can be measured in the urine or blood (see Chapter 5).

- If the body still doesn't get the insulin it needs, then the ketone (acid) level in the body builds up and results in **DKA** (**D**iabetic **K**eto**A**cidosis).

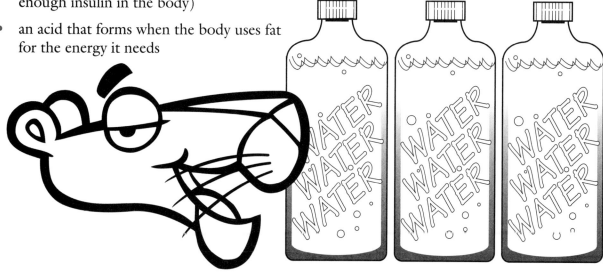

High blood sugar will make you thirsty. Drinking fluids helps "wash-out" ketones.

WHAT ARE THE MAIN CAUSES OF KETONURIA OR OF DKA?

 Forgetting to give one or more insulin shots is the most common cause of DKA in patients with known diabetes. Giving "spoiled" insulin (insulin that got too hot [over 90° F, 32° C] or froze).

 Illness: the amount of insulin usually needs to be increased so the body will have the extra energy from carbohydrates needed to fight the illness. Otherwise, fat is broken down to provide energy.

 Not enough insulin (dose too small).

An insulin pump that is not delivering insulin (usually due to kinked, obstructed or dislodged infusion catheter).

Traumatic stress on the body (particularly type 2 diabetes).

DKA can be very dangerous. It usually does not occur unless large urine ketones or blood ketones (above 3.0 mmol/L) have been present for several hours. It usually occurs in people with known diabetes who forget to check blood or urine ketones as instructed (see below).

WHAT SHOULD BE DONE TO PREVENT DKA?

check for blood or urine ketones (see methods in Chapter 5):

- any time the morning blood/CGM glucose level is above 240 mg/dL (13.3 mmol/L)

- any time the blood/CGM glucose level is above 300 mg/dL (16.7 mmol/L) at any time of day

- with any illness (even vomiting one time)

Call the diabetes care provider immediately if urine ketones are found to be moderate or large or if the blood ketones are above 1.0 mmol/L.

When moderate or large urine ketones or blood ketones (above 1.0 mmol/L) are found, extra rapid-acting insulin is given (by shot if using an insulin pump) every two to three hours to help stop ketones from being made.

The family should then make repeat calls every two hours to the doctor or nurse. Extra doses of rapid-acting insulin will be needed every two hours until the high blood ketones or the moderate or large urine ketones are gone.

It is also important to drink extra liquids. The extra liquids help to wash out the ketones.

It is best **NOT** to exercise as the ketone level may increase.

It is important to keep the blood/CGM glucose level up so that enough insulin can be given to turn off ketone production without having low blood sugar.

People taking metformin (Glucophage) should stop this medicine until the illness is over.

We have found that DKA can be prevented 95% of the time if the instructions in this chapter are followed.

WHAT ARE THE SIGNS OF DKA?

- Usually the blood/CGM glucose level is high. High sugars cause thirst and frequent urination.

- A stomachache, vomiting, or a sweet odor to the breath can occur with high ketones.

- If large urine ketones or blood ketones above 3.0 mmol/L have been present for many hours, deep or troubled breathing can occur. This is a sign to go to the emergency room.

High blood/CGM glucose levels will make you go to the bathroom more often.

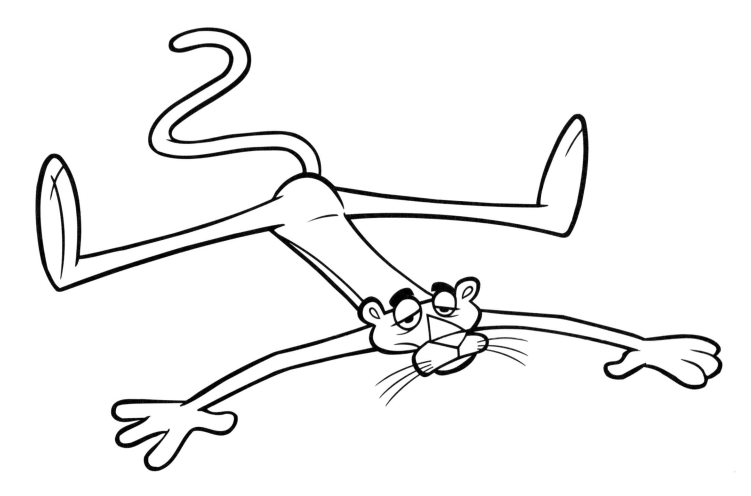

Check your ketones before calling your doctor
when you aren't feeling well.

Chapter 16

Sick-Day and Surgery Management

SICK-DAY MANAGEMENT

People with diabetes get sick just like other people. For example, the average child gets eight colds a year. These may affect the diabetes. Use of the continuous glucose monitor (CGM) can be very helpful during times of illness.

🐾 **It is important to:**

- Always check **urine and/or ketones** and the **blood/CGM glucose levels** with any illness. Check ketones even if the blood/CGM glucose level is normal.

- Call your doctor or nurse if the urine ketone result is moderate or large or if the blood ketone level (using the Precision Xtra™ meter) is above 1.0 mmol/L.

- The earlier you treat the ketones with extra Humalog/NovoLog/Apidra or Regular insulin and fluids, the less chance you will have to go into the hospital.

🐾 **Insulin:**

- If vomiting is present and ketones are negative, the insulin dose may have to be lowered, but **some insulin must be given**.

- If the person vomits three or more times, some doctors will prescribe a Phenergan suppository (or skin-application) or orally dissolved tablets called Zofran® (Table 1). Children under two years of age should not use a Phenergan suppository.

🐾 **Low-Dose Glucagon:**

- Glucagon can be mixed and given with an insulin syringe just like insulin.

- A low dose may be helpful when the blood sugar is low and vomiting continues (see Chapter 6).

- The dose of glucagon is much lower than the dose given for severe hypoglycemia.

- The dose is one unit for every year of age up to 15 units.

- It should not be given if urine ketones are moderate or large (or blood ketones above 1.0 mmol/L).

- Call your doctor or nurse before giving the glucagon injection if you have questions. It can be repeated every 20 minutes if needed.

- Suggestions for sick-day foods are given in Table 2.

- Many medications have a warning label that a person with diabetes should not use the medicine. This is because they may raise the blood/CGM glucose levels a few points.

  - Our view is that if the medicine is needed, go ahead and take it. We can always adjust the insulin if needed.

  - Steroids (e.g., prednisone) are the most difficult (often used for asthma) and, if prescribed, the diabetes care provider should be notified.

- **Type 2 Diabetes:**

  Youth with type 2 diabetes must also remember to check the urine and/or blood ketone level with any illness.

  - If the person is receiving metformin (Glucophage), the pills should be stopped during the illness.

  - It is usually best to return to insulin shots during the illness.

  - Call your doctor or nurse if you have questions.

SURGERY MANAGEMENT

If surgery is planned:

- Call your diabetes care provider AFTER you find out the time of the surgery and if eating food in usual amounts will be allowed.

- Take your own diabetes supplies with you to the surgery:

  - blood sugar meter and strips, with finger poker (lancet)

  - CGM (if used) and extra sensor

  - insulin and syringes

  - glucose (dextrose) tablets or gel

  - blood ketone strips and meter or urine Ketostix

  - glucagon emergency kit

  - if on a pump, equipment to change infusion set if needed

- Take your phone card with your diabetes care provider's numbers.

- If you receive a basal insulin (e.g., by insulin pump or by Lantus or Levemir injection), the basal insulin can be continued during the period of surgery. Then restart bolus pump therapy or bolus insulin injections when the person is able to eat.

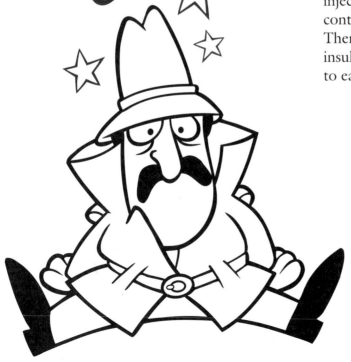

Table 1
Management of Vomiting (Without Ketones)

Avoid solid foods until the vomiting has stopped.

If vomiting is frequent, some doctors recommend giving a Phenergan suppository (or skin application) or an orally dissolved tablet called Zofran, to reduce vomiting. It may be best to wait to give fluids for an hour until the medicine is working. Children under two years of age should not use a Phenergan suppository.

If you do not have an anti-vomiting medication, ask for a prescription at the time of your clinic visit.

Gradually start liquids (juice, Pedialyte®, water, etc.) in small amounts. Juices (especially orange) replace the salts that are lost with vomiting or diarrhea. Pedialyte popsicles are also available.

* Start with a tablespoon of liquid every 10-20 minutes.

* If the blood/CGM glucose level is below 100 mg/dL (5.5 mmol/L), sugar pop or other liquids containing sugar can be given.

* If the blood/CGM glucose level is below 70 mg/dL (3.9 mmol/L) and the person is vomiting, give a low dose of glucagon just as you would give insulin. The dose is 1 unit per year of age up to 15 units (see text). Repeat doses can be given every 20 minutes as needed.

* If the blood/CGM glucose level is above 150 mg/dL (8.3 mmol/L), do not give pop with sugar in it.

* If there is no further vomiting, gradually increase the amount of fluid.

* If vomiting restarts, it may again be necessary to rest the stomach for another hour and then restart the small amounts of fluids. A repeat Phenergan suppository or Zofran tablet can be given after three or four hours.

After a few hours without vomiting, gradually return to a normal diet. Soups are often helpful to start with and they provide needed nutrients.

Table 2
Sick-Day Foods

1 Liquids*

- Fruit juice: apple, cranberry, grape, grapefruit, orange, pineapple, etc.

- Sugar-containing beverages: regular 7Up®, ginger ale, orange juice, cola, PEPSI®, etc.*

- Fruit-flavored drinks: regular Kool-Aid®, lemonade, Hi-C®, etc.*

- Sports drinks: Gatorade®, POWERADE®, etc., any flavor

- Tea with honey or sugar (children less than one year of age should NOT receive honey)

- Pedialyte®, or Infalyte® (especially for younger children)

- JELL-O®: regular (for infants, liquid JELL-O warmed in a bottle) or diet

- Popsicles, regular or diet

- Broth-type soup: bouillon, chicken noodle soup, Cup-a-Soup®

2 Solids (when ready)

- Saltine crackers

- Banana (or other fruit)

- Applesauce

- Bread or toast

- Graham crackers

- Soup

***Sugar-free may be needed depending on blood/CGM glucose levels (e.g., greater than 150 mg/dL [8.3 mmol/L]).**

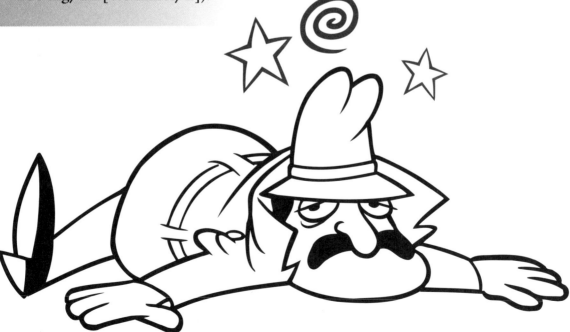

Table 3
Sick-Day Management:
When/Who to Call for Emergency Care

- If you have vomited more than three times and can keep nothing in your stomach, and urine ketones are not moderate or large or blood ketones above 1.0 mmol/L, call your primary care physician.

- *If help is needed with an insulin dose, call your diabetes care provider.*

- If moderate or large ketones are present or blood ketones are above 1.0 mmol/L, call your diabetes care provider.

- If you have difficulty breathing or have "deep breathing," you need to go to an emergency room immediately. This usually indicates severe acidosis (ketoacidosis).

- Low blood sugar (hypoglycemia):

If there is any unusual behavior such as confusion, slurred speech, double vision, inability to move or talk, or jerking, someone should give sugar or instant glucose. Glucagon (Chapter 6) is given if the person is unconscious or if a convulsion (seizure) occurs. The diabetes care provider should be contacted if a severe reaction occurs. In case of a convulsion or loss of consciousness, it may be necessary to call the paramedics or to go to an emergency room. Have an emergency number posted by the phone.

Your insulin dose may change when you are sick, but you always need some insulin.

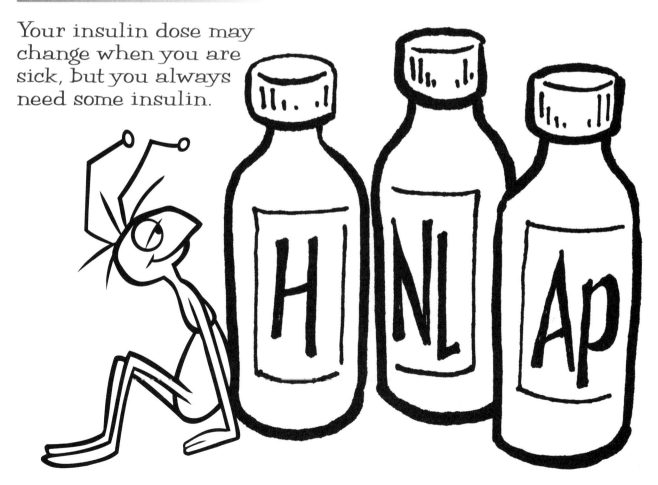

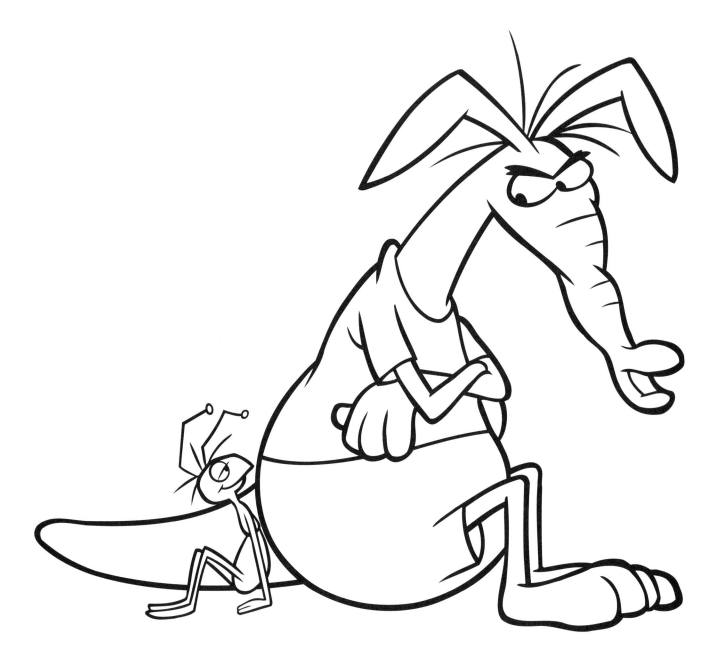

Family support is very important
for the person with diabetes.

Chapter 17
Family Concerns

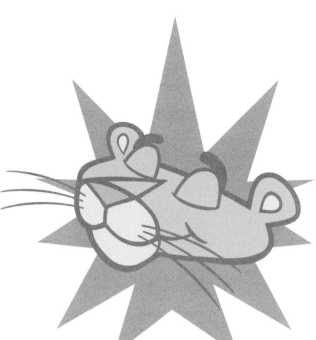

Diabetes is a family disease. This means that all family members must help. The people who do best with their diabetes have the help and support of all family members.

 It is important for children with diabetes to be treated just like other children. A rule to follow is:

THINK OF THE CHILD FIRST AND THEN THE DIABETES.

It is important that all family members share their feelings (see Chapter 10).

Siblings often feel left out when the child with diabetes needs more attention.

This should be discussed with the other children and time should be set aside for them as well.

Perhaps the most supportive and loving act that parents, brothers and sisters can make for the person with diabetes is to remove high-sugar foods (candy, sugar pop, donuts, cookies, etc.) from the home. These foods have little nutritional value. If they are around, they may be eaten without taking extra insulin, which will raise the blood/CGM glucose values.

SPECIFIC AREAS OF CONCERN

1. The stress of the diagnosis of diabetes is real for all family members.

   One of the four big influences on blood sugar levels is stress (see Chapter 14). The social worker or psychologist is available to help in dealing with stress.

2. Extra activity and excitement may cause a low blood sugar in people with diabetes. Some of the following may include delayed meals as well as increased activity:

   * family picnics
   * sleepovers
   * trips to the beach or hiking
   * school field days or trips
   * a trip to Disney® or other theme parks
   * special days such as Christmas or Hanukkah

Thinking ahead, reducing the insulin dose, doing more blood/CGM glucose levels and giving extra snacks may result in a better day for everyone. Wearing an ID bracelet is particularly important on trips.

Needle fears occur in about one-fourth of all people. The psychosocial team may be helpful, particularly in suggesting distractions (TV, toys, books) or relaxation techniques. The use of the Insuflon or I-Port (Chapter 9) is also sometimes helpful.

 Missed shots (or insulin boluses for the pumper) result in an elevated HbA1c level and an increased risk for diabetic complications. Help from other family members, teachers, friends or counselors may be needed.

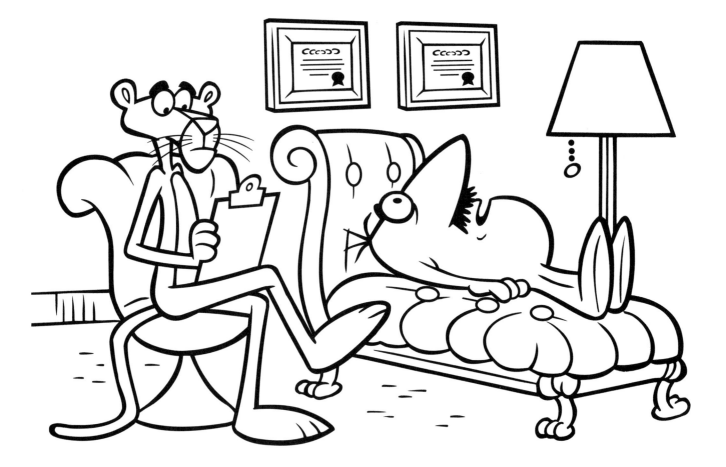

Social workers and psychologists
are there to help you.

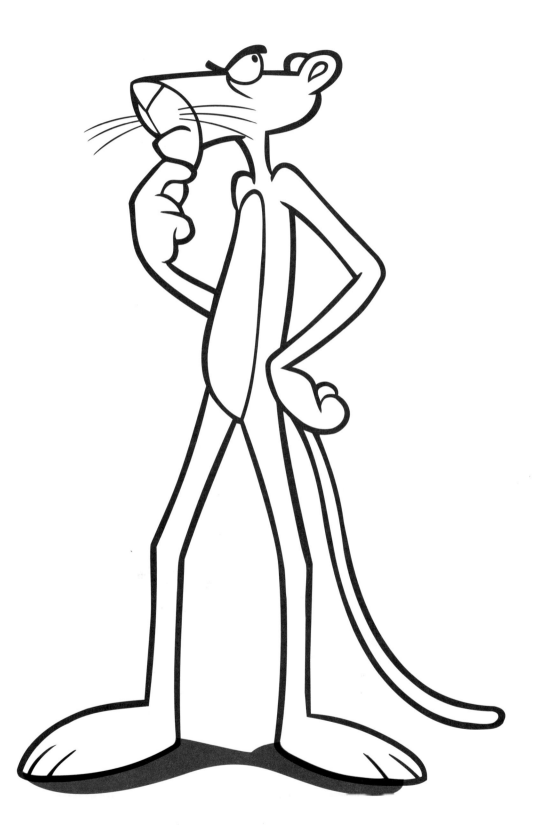

Think of the person first
and THEN the diabetes.

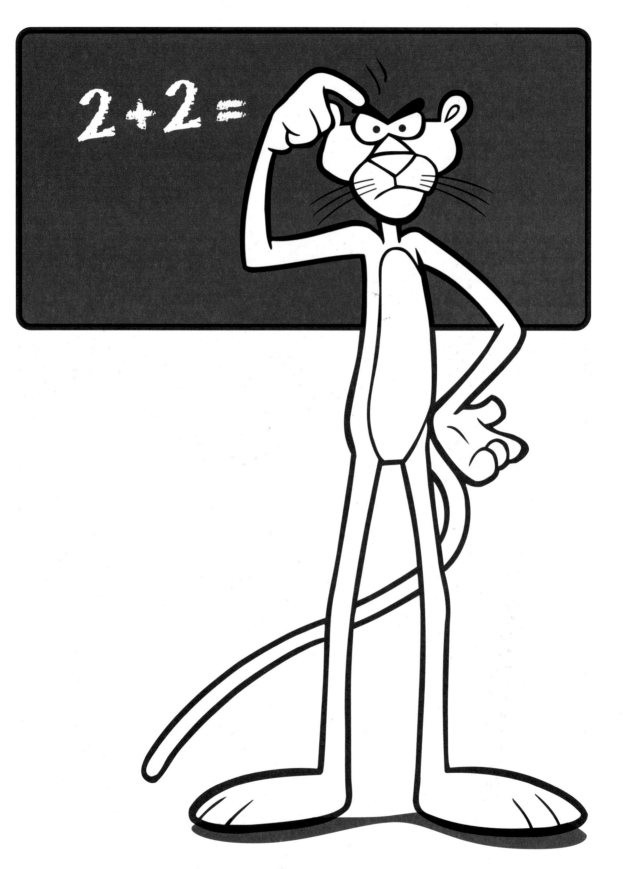

High or low blood sugars
may affect school performance.

Chapter 18
Care of Children at Different Ages

Children of different ages are able to handle different tasks and responsibilities. These may vary from day to day and week to week. This is true for diabetes-related tasks and non-diabetes tasks. It can be helpful for family members to have an idea of what to expect at different ages.

(See the tables of age-responsibilities in *"Understanding Diabetes"*, Chapter 18.)

Below age 8 years

* Parents do all tasks.

* Children gradually learn to cooperate.

* Shots are often given after meals or snacks (to vary the dose) depending upon what was eaten.

Ages 8-12 years

* Children begin to give some of their own shots. A common mistake is to push for too much responsibility before the child is ready.

* Having a friend spend the night or staying at a friend's house often begins during this period. As the children are often very active and use more energy from staying

up later than usual, it is best to reduce the insulin dose.

* At this age, fine motor control and the sense of accuracy needed to draw up the insulin develops.

* It is important to continue to check doses of insulin drawn by the child and the blood/CGM glucose devices to review their readings.

* The idea of maintaining optimal sugar control to prevent later diabetes complications can initially be understood around age 12 or 13 years.

Ages 13-18 years

One of the most difficult chores for many teens is writing the blood sugar values in a log book (or downloading CGM results). It is important to do this or trends in blood/CGM glucose values will be missed. Often the parents agree to do this (with the teen's OK). It is also a way for the parents to stay involved with the diabetes care and to step back in if blood/CGM glucose levels are not being done.

WHAT IS THE AGE WHEN SELF-CARE SHOULD HAPPEN?

- Children should be encouraged to assume self-care as they are able.

- There isn't a "magic" age when children should take over everything.

- If too much is expected too soon, feelings of failure and low self-esteem with poor diabetes self-care may result.

- **It is now believed that a supportive adult can be valuable for any person with diabetes, no matter their age.**

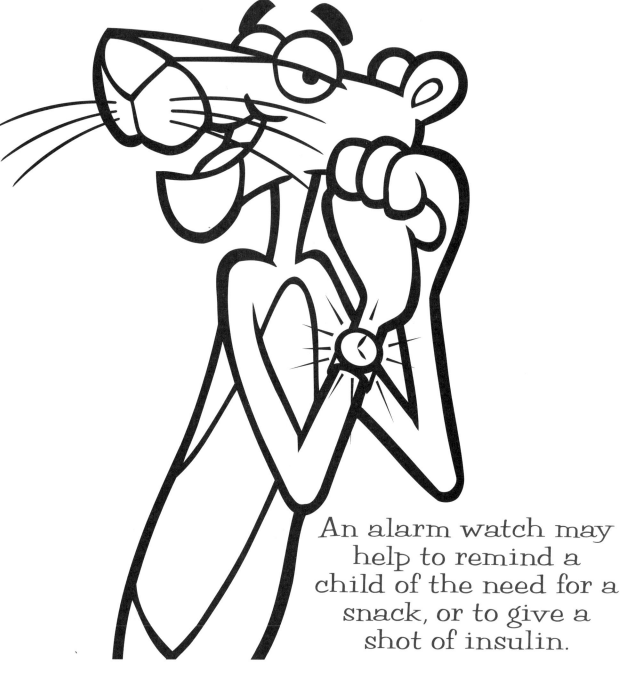

An alarm watch may help to remind a child of the need for a snack, or to give a shot of insulin.

Children between the ages of 8-12 can begin to help manage their diabetes.

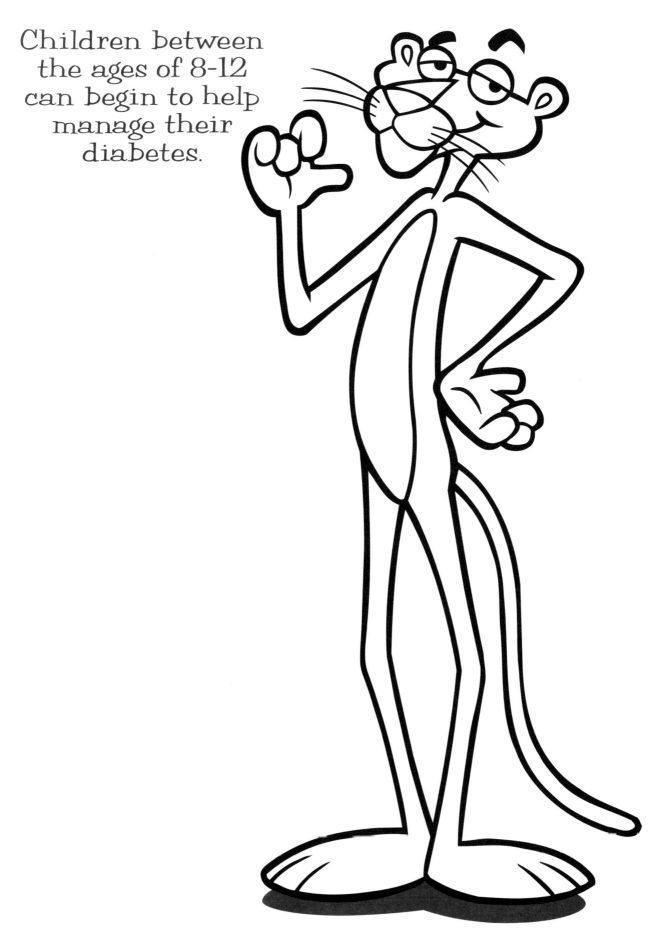

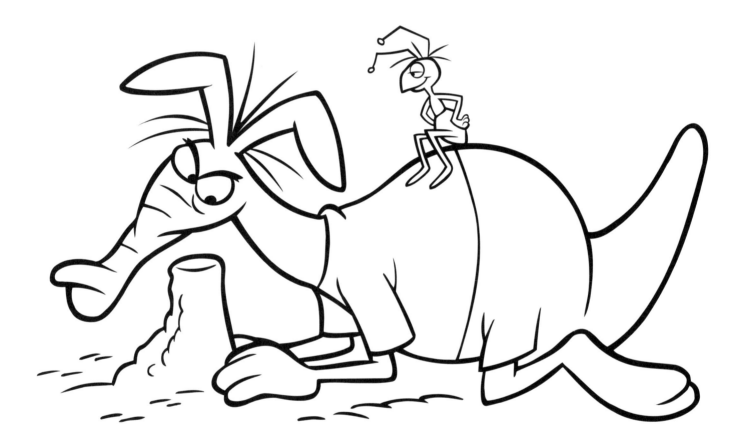

Chapter 19

Diabetes Management in the Toddler/ Preschooler

Chapter 18 deals with traits related and not-related to diabetes for different aged children, including toddlers and preschoolers. Because this is the age-group in which diabetes is increasing the most rapidly, it was decided that further details relating to management might be helpful.

BASAL-BOLUS INSULIN THERAPY (also see Chapter 8)

When possible, basal-bolus insulin therapy should be used in this aged child. The use of NPH insulin is more apt to result in low blood/CGM glucose levels, particularly during the night.

The two basal insulins are Lantus™ or Levemir™. They are usually given once daily, preferably in the morning. Then if activity does not last a full 24 hours, insulin activity is less in the early morning hours when lows are worrisome. Some parents give the injection (often in the buttocks) while the child is still asleep.

The preferred bolus insulin is Humalog™, Novalog™or Aprida™. In contrast to older children, the shot is often given after the meal since eating can be unpredictable in this age group. The dose can then be chosen after seeing what the child eats. Blood/CGM glucose levels will be higher after meals in comparison to giving the bolus 15 to 20 minutes before the meal. However, the goals for blood/CGM glucose levels (100-200 mg/dL or 5.5-11.1 mmol/L) and for HbA1c levels (7.5 to 8.5%) are not as strict for this age group in comparison to older children.

Use of the I-Port or Insuflon (Chapter 9) may help children who are having difficulty with injections.

Smaller (3ml) vials of Humalog can be ordered from pharmacies. The NDC number (to tell the pharmacist) is 002-7510-17. Hopefully, the co-pay will also be less.

INSULIN PUMPS

An advantage of insulin pumps in this age-group is that frequent shots are avoided. Several studies have shown that insulin pumps are safe in children this age. The parents obviously do all of the pump management and must agree on wanting the pump for their child. In some parents, early pump use has been associated with more stress, although this usually lessens with time. The use of temporary basal rates for periods of high activity or at the time of low blood/CGM glucose values can be advantageous. HbA1c levels usually do not show change with pump use in this aged child. Thus, the major reasons for pump use are safety and convenience.

CONTINUOUS GLUCOSE MONITORS (CGM)

As with pumps, a CGM can be used in this age group **when the family is ready**. Safety may be enhanced with the alarms for high and low glucose levels. The CGM provides convenience for the parents being able to see the glucose levels and in not having to do as many finger, toe or heel pokes for blood sugar levels. Some blood sugars will still be necessary, however. The major drawback is adequate "real-estate", especially if also using an insulin pump. The diabetes nurse educator can help to explore this issue.

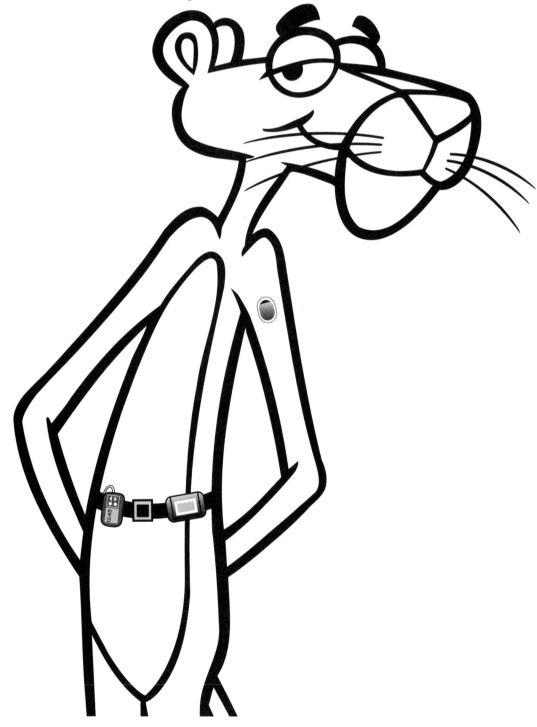

Chapter 20

Special Challenges of the Teen Years

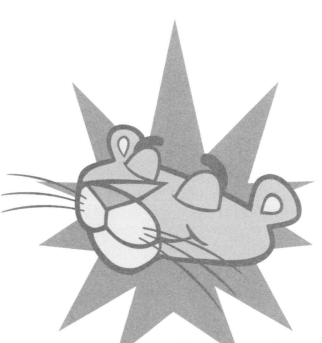

The teen years are a time when young people go between wanting to be an independent adult and wanting to stay a dependent child. It is not surprising that they go back and forth when it comes to taking over the diabetes responsibilities. Many research studies now show that when parents stay involved in diabetes management, the diabetes will be in better control.

THE CHALLENGES

- The teen-aged years are often the most difficult for having optimal sugar control (including a HbA1c value below 7.5 percent [see Chapter 14]). And yet, they are important years in relation to an increased risk for diabetes complications.

- Growth and sex hormones are at high levels and interfere with insulin activity.

- Insulin pumps, more frequent insulin shots or boluses, and the basal insulins, insulin glargine (Lantus) or insulin detemir (Levemir) can help some teens. However, if meal and snack shots (or boluses for pumpers) are missed, the HbA1c will be high.

- Driving a car safely is very important beginning in the teen years. It is important to check a blood/CGM glucose level before driving. Driving with a low blood sugar can result in problems that can be just as severe as if driving while drunk.

- Diabetes is often not a priority to the teenager. Teenagers have special issues including:

  - **struggle for independence**

  - **growth and body changes**

  - **self-identity**

  - **sports activities (see Chapter 13)**

  - **peer relationships**

  - **sexuality**

  - **consistency:** is considered a key word in diabetes management. This refers to eating, exercise, stress, doing blood/CGM glucose levels or times of insulin shots/boluses. It is often hard for teens to be consistent.

  - **driving a car**

  - **college**

  - **emotional changes**

These are all discussed in detail in the 12th edition of "Understanding Diabetes".

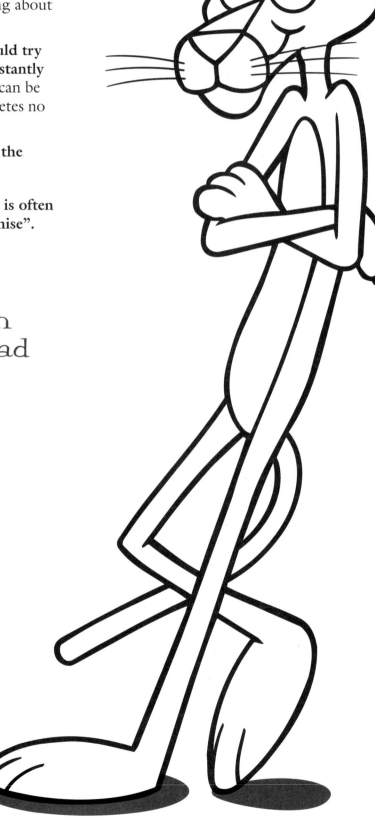

❀ **Parents must:**

- **find ways to stay involved in diabetes management.** They can be helpful in keeping the log book, downloading meters or CGMs and in talking about insulin dosage.

- **be available to help, but should try not to be overbearing or constantly nagging.** A supportive adult can be helpful for a person with diabetes no matter their age.

- **help with communication to the diabetes care providers.**

It is not surprising that diabetes is often referred to as a "disease of compromise".

Teenagers with diabetes can lead normal lives.

Normal teen activities can provide much-needed exercise

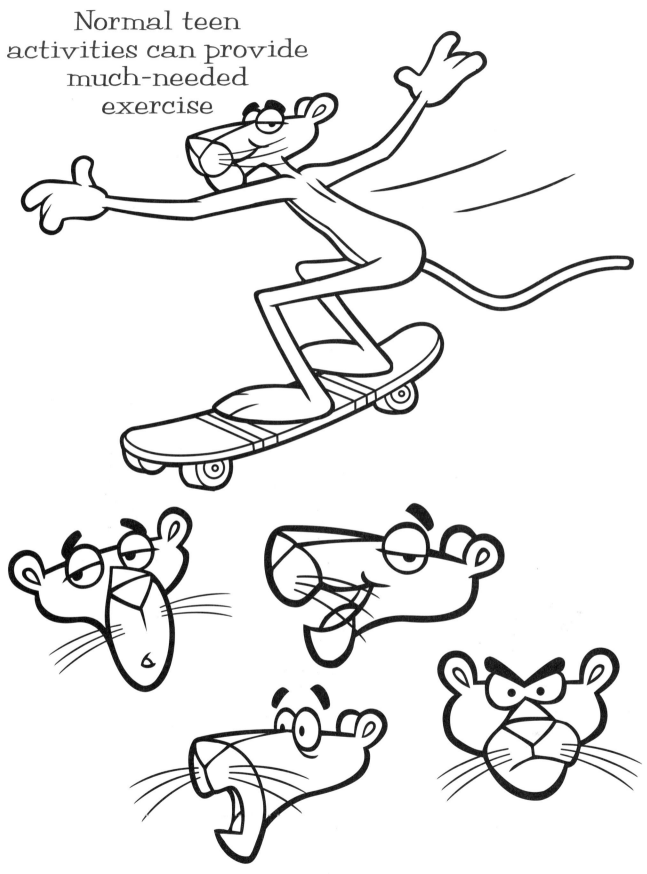

Teenagers have their own special challenges.

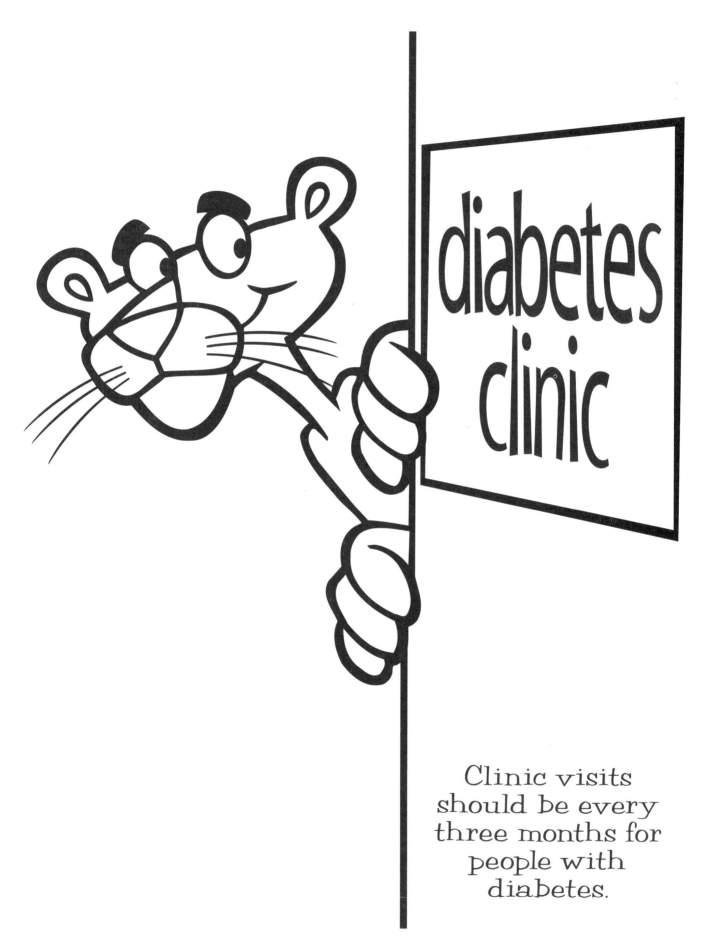

diabetes
clinic

Clinic visits
should be every
three months for
people with
diabetes.

Chapter 21

Outpatient Management, Education, Support Groups and Standards of Care

WHAT SHOULD HAPPEN AFTER A DIAGNOSIS OF DIABETES?

* Regular follow-up visits should be every three months for people with diabetes. Diabetes education should continue for the patient and family at these visits.

* The insulin dose may be changed during these visits. It is usually increased one-half unit per pound of weight gained (just to have the same dose for weight).

* Growth and other signs of sugar control such as liver size and finger curvatures are checked. If blood/CGM glucose values are high, the sugar collects on the joint proteins and finger curvatures may result.

* On the physical exam, thyroid size and eye changes are checked.

* The HbA1c level (see Chapter 14) should be done every three months.

* After having diabetes for three years as a teen or adult, eye exams by an eye doctor and urine microalbumin levels to check the kidneys, are very important to have each year (see Chapter 23).

* For people with type 2 diabetes, the eye and kidney evaluations should be done at the time of diagnosis, and then yearly.

WHAT ELSE IS IMPORTANT?

* Communication (fax, email) of blood/CGM glucose values to the health care provider is often helpful.

* The families should let their diabetes provider or diabetes team know about any of the following:

  * any severe low blood sugar (hypoglycemic) reactions

  * frequent mild reactions

  * moderate or large urine ketones or blood ketones above 1.0 mmol/L

  * any planned surgery

  * if at least half of the blood/CGM glucose values are not in the desired range for age (see Chapter 7)

* Support groups and special educational programs (Research Updates, Carb Counting Class, Pump or CGM classes, Grandparents Workshop, College-Bound Workshop, etc.) are available in many areas.

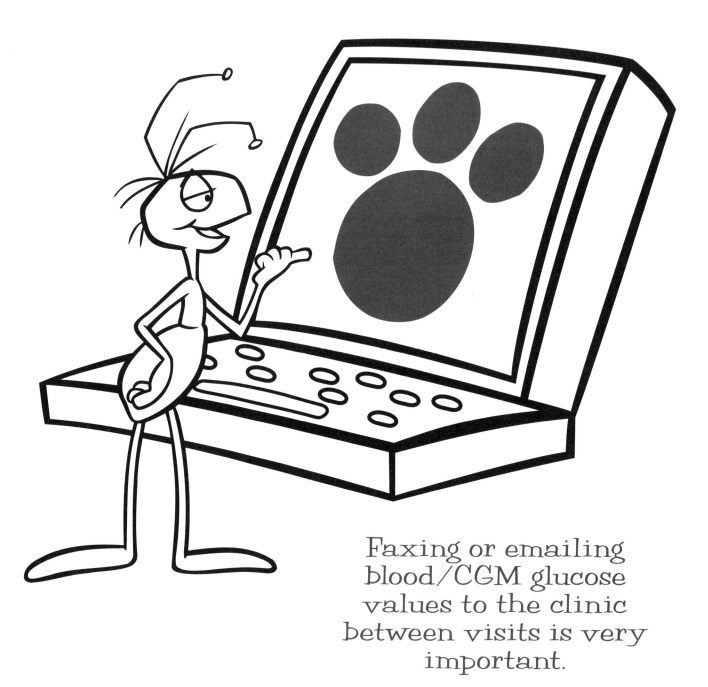

✿ Special events (family workshops, bike trips, camps, a Halloween party, etc.) help children and families to learn more about diabetes. They also provide a chance to talk to others who have a family member with diabetes.

Faxing or emailing blood/CGM glucose values to the clinic between visits is very important.

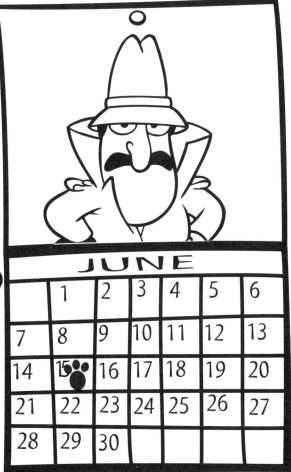

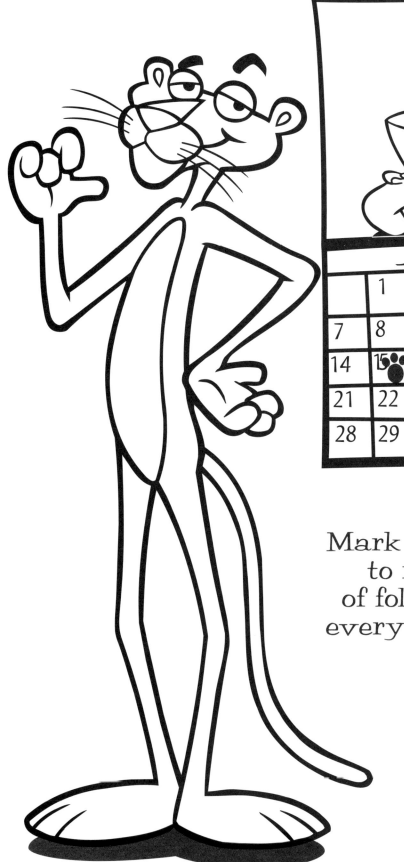

Mark your calendar
to remind you
of follow-up visits
every three months.

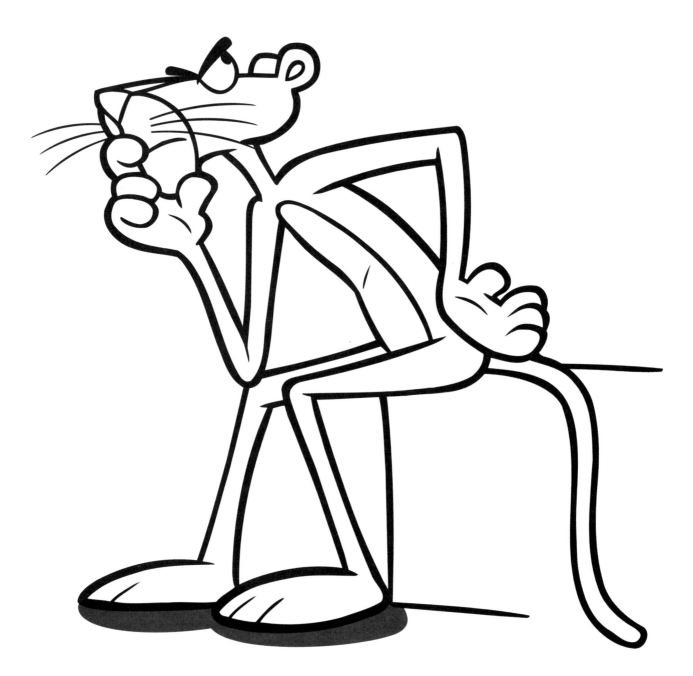

You need to think about your insulin dose.

Chapter 22
Adjusting the Insulin Dosage and "Thinking" Scales

Six to twelve months after the diagnosis of diabetes, many families feel OK with changing the insulin doses on their own.

HOW AND WHEN SHOULD AN INSULIN DOSE BE CHANGED?

1. Looking at blood/CGM glucose patterns over the last week:

🐾 It is necessary to know which insulin is acting at the time of the highs or lows in order to make the correct changes (see figures in Chapter 8).

🐾 If more than half of the blood/CGM glucose values at any time of the day are above the desired range for the age of the person (see table in Chapter 7):

- The insulin dose acting at the time of the high blood/CGM glucose values should be increased.

- If values are still high after three days, the dose can be increased again.

🐾 If there are more than two lows (below 60 mg/dL [3.3 mmol/L]) at one time of day:

- The insulin dose acting at that time should be decreased.

- If more lows occur, the dose can be decreased again the next day.

🐾 With small children, the change in dose may be by one half to one unit.

🐾 With older children and teens, the change in dose may be by one or two units.

🐾 Tables are given in the larger book, *"Understanding Diabetes"* (Chapter 22) for people wanting more detailed suggestions on changing insulin doses for high or low blood/CGM glucose values.

2. Using a "correction factor":

🐾 Most people use a combination of a **"correction factor"** and **carbohydrate (carb) counting** (see Chapter 12) to determine the total dose of rapid-acting insulin before meals and snacks.

🐾 The **correction factor** can be used to "correct" a high blood sugar down to a **target blood/CGM glucose level** (e.g., 150 mg/dL [8.3 mmol/L] during the night and 120 mg/dL [6.7 mmol] during the day).

The most common **correction factor** is to give one unit of insulin for every 50 mg/dL (2.8 mmol/L) of glucose above 150 mg/dL (8.3 mmol/L), e.g., if the blood/CMG glucose level is 250 mg/dL (13.9 mmol/L), the correction factor is 2 units. Many teens and adults correct down to 120 mg/dL (6.7 mmol/L) or even 100 mg/dL (5.5 mmol/L) during the day. However, every person is different and the **correction factor** should be adjusted to fit the individual.

At bedtime, during the night, or before exercise, the correction factor may be reduced by half.

It is generally wise to wait two hours between correction insulin dosages.

3. Using "thinking" scales:

The insulin dose is figured by considering many factors, including:

- the blood/CGM glucose level
- illness
- any exercise that has been or is to be done
- stress
- food to be eaten
- menses

4. Changes for Lantus or Levemir:

Adjustments are usually made based on the morning (fasting) blood/CGM glucose levels.

Doses are increased or decreased if blood/CGM glucose levels are above or below the recommended values for age (see Chapter 7).

As suggested above, dose changes for a young child may be by one half to one unit, and for older children (and teens), by one to two units.

Suggested waiting times between dose changes are 3-4 days unless blood/CGM glucose values are <70 or >300 mg/dL (<3.9 or >16.7 mmol/L).

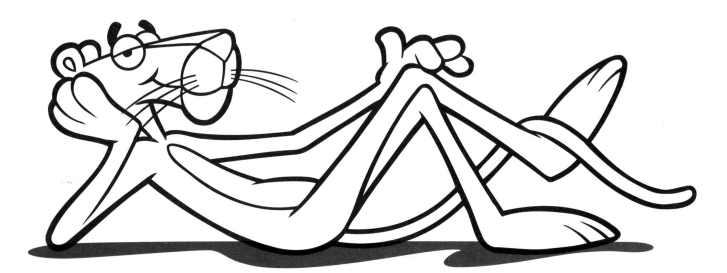

Table
Example of Insulin Adjustments

Blood Sugar		Correction Factor*	Carbohydrates**		Total Units
mg/dL	mmol/L	Units of Insulin	(grams of carbs)	Units of Insulin	of Insulin
Less than 150	8.3	0	(15g)	1	1
200	11.1	1	(30g)	2	3
250	13.9	2	(45g)	3	5
300	16.7	3	(60g)	4	7
350	19.4	4	(75g)	5	9

*Assuming a correction factor of 1 unit of rapid-acting insulin per 50 mg/dL (2.8 mmol/L) above 150 mg/dL (8.3 mmol/L).

**In this example, 1 unit of insulin is given for each 15g of carbs. The carbs are increased by 15g for each line in the table.

The insulin doses and the amount of food eaten may need to change with sports activities.

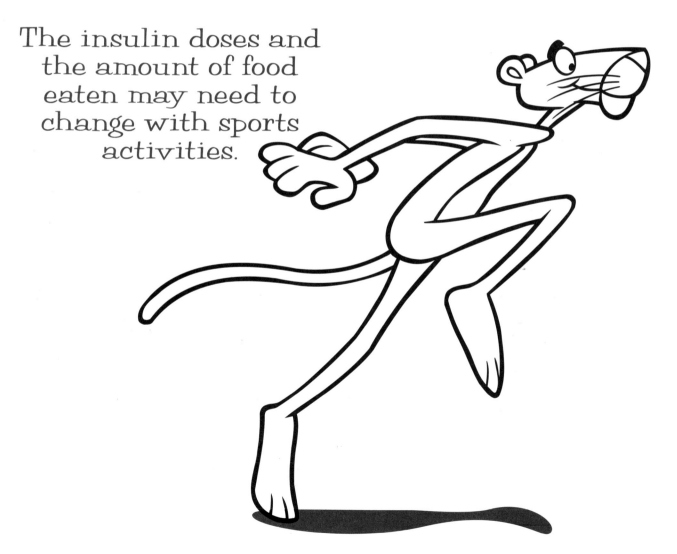

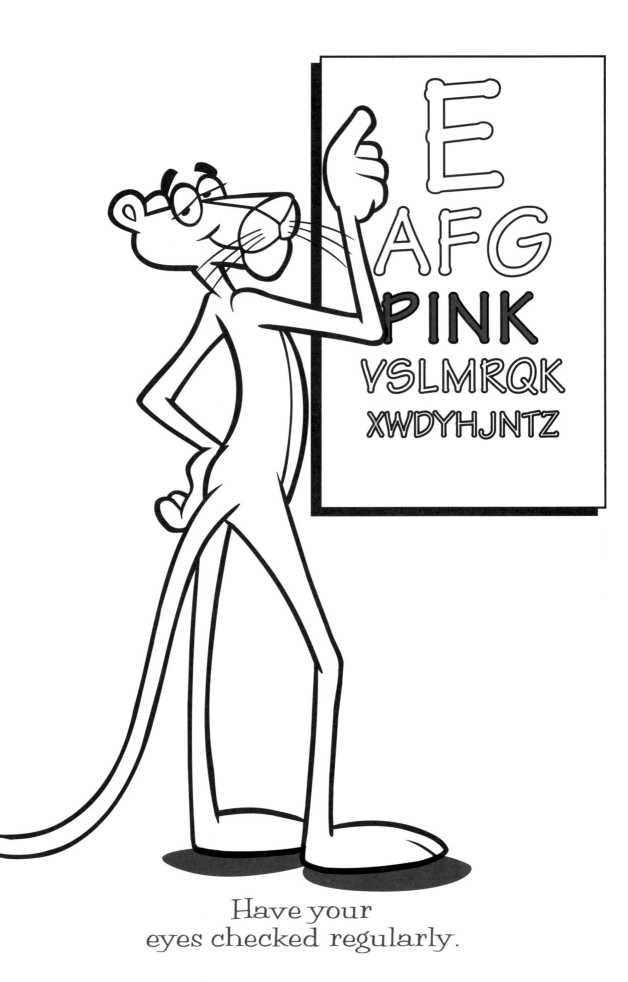

Have your
eyes checked regularly.

Chapter 23

Long-term Complications of Diabetes

WHAT CAN MAKE THE RISK OF THESE COMPLICATIONS LESS?

🐾 Optimal blood sugar control will reduce the risk for eye, kidney, nerve, and heart complications of diabetes by more than 50 percent as shown by the DCCT (Chapter 14).

🐾 Not smoking (or chewing) tobacco also helps.

🐾 Other factors are blood pressure and cholesterol. Researchers at our Center showed that even mild increases in blood pressure are dangerous for the eyes and kidneys.

HOW ARE COMPLICATIONS FOUND?

Small Blood Vessels (Eyes and Kidneys):

- Eye exams (and especially photographs) by the eye doctor tell if someone is developing eye damage.

- The urine microalbumin determination tells if someone is getting early kidney damage at a time when it may still be reversible. The instructions for doing the

microalbumin level to detect early kidney damage are at the end of Chapter 23 in *"Understanding Diabetes"*. We prefer overnight urine collections because a false positive result is less likely.

- Screening for the eyes (eye exam) and kidneys (urine microalbumins) should be done once yearly for people who have had type 1 diabetes for three or more years and have reached puberty (age 10 to 12 years).

- People who have type 2 diabetes should have the eye and kidney evaluations done soon after diagnosis and then every year.

- Families may need to help remind the health care team that it is time to do the annual microalbumin screen or to see an eye doctor.

- The most important treatment of early eye or kidney damage is improving sugar control.

- Treatment of early kidney damage is also done by lowering blood pressure. A blood pressure medicine called an ACE-inhibitor is often helpful.

- If many eye changes are present, laser treatment to the back of the eye (retina) may help to prevent more severe problems.

Large Blood Vessel Problems in Adults (Heart and Blood Vessels):

- Heart attacks and other blood vessel diseases are a greater risk in adults with diabetes.

- Cholesterol levels and a lipid panel should be checked yearly.

- A baby aspirin (in adults) and/or a fish oil capsule (omega-3 fatty acid) taken once or twice daily may help in prevention.

- Adult diabetes clinics usually do special evaluations of the heart (EKG's) and blood vessels at regular intervals.

Finger curvatures
can be a sign of
high blood/CGM glucose
levels over many years.

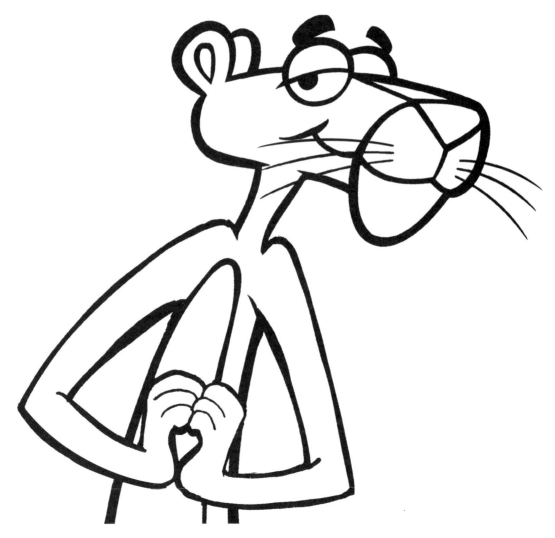

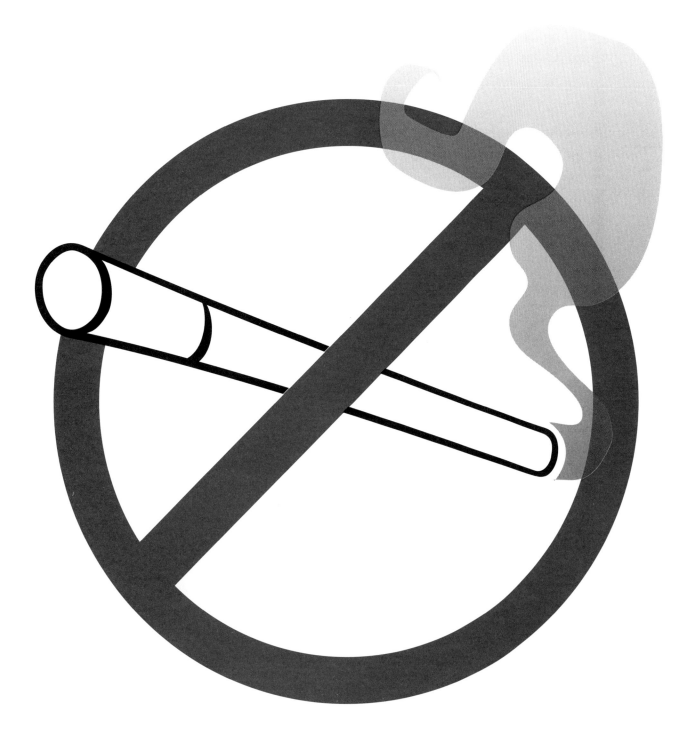

DO NOT SMOKE!
(or chew tobacco!)

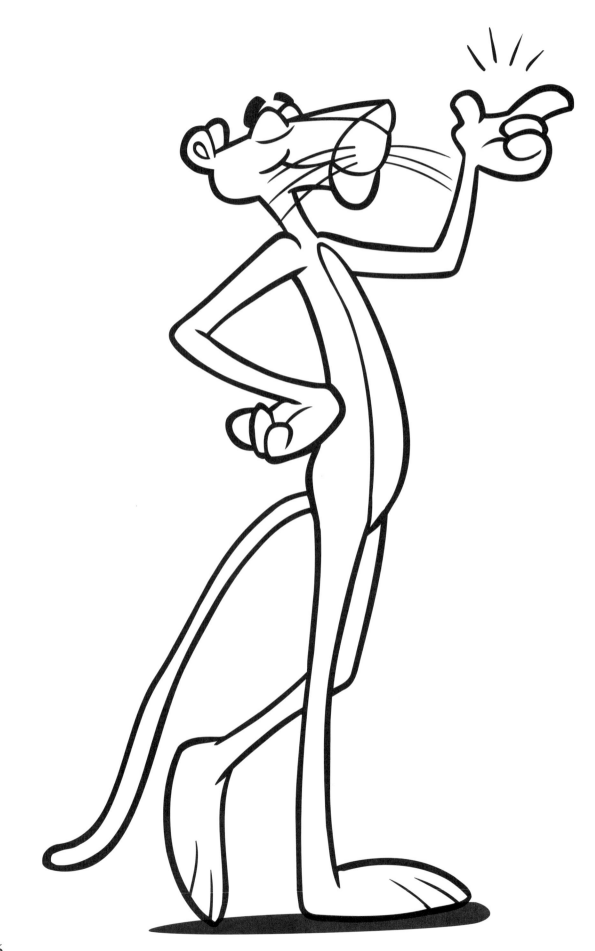

Chapter 24
Associated Autoimmune Conditions of Type 1 Diabetes

Other autoimmune (self-allergy) diseases are also associated with type 1 diabetes. This is due to the inheritance of genes increasing the risk for autoimmunity. Three examples of autoimmune diseases seen more frequently in people with type 1 diabetes are discussed below.

AUTOIMMUNE DISEASES THAT CAN OCCUR IN PEOPLE WITH DIABETES:

🐾 **Thyroid problems:** thyroid problems (like type 1 diabetes) are due to autoimmunity (see Chapter 3). Antibodies are made against the thyroid gland. About 1 in 20 people with diabetes need treatment and this can be with a daily thyroid hormone replacement pill.

We recommend careful examination of the thyroid gland with clinic visits every three months. Laboratory evaluations should be done annually, particularly if the thyroid gland is enlarged or if there is any fall-off in height attainment. The TSH (**T**hyroid **S**timulating **H**ormone) is the best laboratory value for screening, although some physicians also order a blood thyroid hormone level (T4 or Free T4).

🐾 **Celiac disease:** this is an allergy to the wheat protein, gluten. It occurs in approximately 1 of every 20 people with diabetes. There may be stomach complaints (pain, gas, diarrhea) or poor growth. Half of the people with celiac disease have no symptoms.

We recommend routine screening of all people with diabetes with the blood transglutaminase level (or other assays). If the person with diabetes is positive, other family members should also be screened. The treatment is to remove all wheat, rye and barley products from the diet. Meeting with a dietitian is important. Websites for obtaining more information on celiac disease and foods to avoid are given in Chapter 24 of *"Understanding Diabetes"*.

🐾 **Adrenal disorders:** Autoimmunity against the adrenal gland (Addison's disease) can occur, but is quite rare (1 in 500 people with type 1 diabetes). Cortisol, the hormone the body is unable to produce in Addison's disease, is especially important during stress. It can be treated with hormone replacement pills and is important to diagnose if present.

School Diabetes Management Checklist for Parents

_____ Discuss specific care of your child with the teachers, school nurse, bus driver, coaches and other staff who will be involved.

_____ Complete the individualized school health care plan with the help of the school staff (using the healthcare provider order form from the diabetes team).

_____ Make sure your child understands the details of who will help him/her with blood sugars, shots and treatment of high or low sugars at school and where supplies will be kept. Supplies should be kept in a place where they are always available if needed.

_____ Make arrangements for the school to send home blood sugar records weekly.

_____ Keep current phone numbers where you can be reached. Collect equipment for school: meter, strips and finger-poker, lancets, insulin, insulin syringes or pen, biohazard container, log book or a copy of blood sugar record form, extra insulin pump supplies, urine or blood ketone strips, photo for substitute teacher's folder.

_____ Food and drinks; parents need to check intermittently to make sure supplies are not used up:

▼ juice cans or boxes (approximately 15g of carb each)

▼ glucose tablets

▼ instant glucose or cake decorating gel

▼ crackers (± peanut butter and/or cheese)

▼ quarters to buy sugar pop (soda) if needed

▼ Fruit Roll-Ups

▼ dried fruit

▼ raisins or other snacks

▼ box with the child's name to store these food and drink items

Parents want to know that their child is in safe hands while at school. It is the parents' responsibility (not the child's) to inform and educate the school. Parents also want to make sure their child is not treated differently as a result of having diabetes.

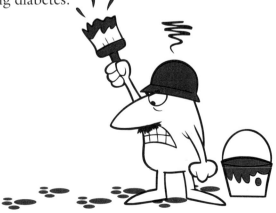

Chapter 25
The School or Work and Diabetes

WHAT SHOULD BE DONE?

🐾 Many schools now require school health plans. The diabetes team initially fills out the "Healthcare Provider Order for Student with Diabetes" (Table 1). An Individualized School Health Plan or **IHP** (Table 2) is then filled out by the parents and the school nurse or aide. You are welcome to copy these forms (Tables 1 and 2).

🐾 The parents must also provide supplies for the school (see School Diabetes Management Checklist for Parents). Some children keep a separate meter and strips at the school. Others bring their home meter and supplies in their backpack.

🐾 Other forms that you may want to copy from the 12th edition of *"Understanding Diabetes"* (Chapter 25) are:

1) Diabetes School Management and Supply Checklist

2) Individualized Health Plan – School Nurse Checklist

3) Insulin Pumps in the School Setting

4) Continuous Glucose Monitoring (CGM) in the School

WHAT CAN HAPPEN AT SCHOOL?

• Low blood sugars are the most likely emergency to occur at school. Treatment is reviewed in the IHP (Table 2). If a child leaves the classroom while having a low blood sugar, they **must** have someone with them. It may be helpful for the family to copy and review the table on mild, moderate and severe reactions with the school (see Chapter 6). *Supplies for treating lows will also need to be provided by the family.*

• High blood sugars and/or ketones may also occur at school, particularly with stress, illness, overeating or lack of exercise. If the blood/CGM glucose level is above 300 mg/dL (16.7 mmol/L) the urine or blood ketones need to be checked. When the blood sugar is high it is generally necessary to go to the bathroom more frequently. Treatments for high blood sugar is reviewed in the IHP (Table 2). *If small to moderate urine ketones or blood ketones above 0.6 mmol/L occur, the parents need to be called.*

Table 1
Healthcare Provider Order for Student with Diabetes

Student: _____ D.O.B.: _____ School _____ Grade _____

Doctor_____ Phone_____ Diabetes Educator_____ Phone _____

Monitor Blood Glucose: ☐ Before Lunch   ☐ After Lunch   ☐ Before PE   ☐ After PE   ☐ Before Snack
☐ Before leaving to get on bus/going home   ☐ As needed for signs/symptoms of low or high blood glucose

Blood glucose at which parent should be notified   Low < _____ mg/dL and High > _____ mg/dL

Target range for blood glucose > _____ mg/dL to < _____ mg/dL

Hypoglycemia Student should not be sent to the office unaccompanied if symptomatic or BS less than 70 mg/dL

- Blood glucose below _____ mg/dL and/or symptomatic: Treat with 10 to 15 gram carbohydrate snack.

- Mild symptoms: Treat with juice, glucose tabs, etc. until above: _____ mg/dL, then snack or lunch.

- Moderate symptoms, if unable to drink juice: Administer glucose gel. Repeat until above: _____ mg/dL, then snack or lunch.

- Severe symptoms, which may include seizures, unconsciousness, unable or unwilling to take gel or juice:
Administer Glucagon _____ mg (_____ cc) subQ or IM if trained staff available and call 911.

Hyperglycemia

- ☐ Check urine ketones if blood glucose is over 300 mg/dL or with symptoms of illness/vomiting. If ketones present, call parents, provide water and student should not exercise. Student may need insulin via injection.

- ☐ Use insulin orders (see below) when blood glucose is _____ mg/dL.

- ☐ Recommend student be released from school when ketones are moderate/large or symptoms of illness in order to be treated and monitored more closely by parent/guardian.

Medication

Student is on ☐ oral diabetes medication(s)   Dose: _____ mg/dL   **Times to be given** _____

Student is on ☐ insulin. Type: _____   Dose: _____ mg/dL   **Times to be given** _____

Blood Glucose Correction and Insulin Dosage using (Rapid Acting) Insulin: _____ units/_____ mg >_____ mg/dL

or: Blood Glucose Range _____mg/dL (_____ mmol/L) Administer _____ units

Blood Glucose Range _____mg/dL (_____ mmol/L) Administer _____ units

Blood Glucose Range _____mg/dL (_____ mmol/L) Administer _____ units and check ketones

Blood Glucose Range _____mg/dL (_____ mmol/L) Administer _____ units and check ketones

Carbohydrate counting _____ unit(s) of insulin per _____ grams of carbohydrate with lunch.

- ☐ Parent/guardian authorized to increase or decrease correction within the following range: +/– 2 units of insulin

- ☐ Parent/guardian authorized to increase or decrease insulin to carbohydrate ratio within the following range: 1 unit per prescribed grams of carbohydrates +/– 5 grams of carbohydrates.

Student's Self Care (ability level to be determined by school nurse and parent with input from healthcare provider)

Totally independent management.........................☐ Yes ☐ No	Self injects with trained staff supervision.................☐ Yes ☐ No	
(If independent, complete self-management agreement)	Injections to be done by trained staff.....................☐ Yes ☐ No	
Needs verification of blood glucose by staff..........☐ Yes ☐ No	Self treats mild hypoglycemia ....☐ Yes ☐ No	
Assist/testing to be done by trained staff..............☐ Yes ☐ No	Monitors own snacks and meals..............................☐ Yes ☐ No	
Administers insulin independently ....☐ Yes ☐ No	Independently counts carbohydrates........................☐ Yes ☐ No	
Self injects with verification of dose ....☐ Yes ☐ No	Monitors and interprets urine/blood ketones..........☐ Yes ☐ No	

SIGNATURES

My signature below provides authorization for the above written orders and exchange of health information to assist the school nurse in developing an Individualized Health Plan. I understand that all procedures will be implemented in accordance with state laws and regulations and may be performed by unlicensed designated school personnel under the training and supervision provided by the school nurse. This order is for a maximum of one year.

Physician_____   Date _____

Parent_____   Date _____

School Nurse _____   Date _____

Table 2
Individualized Health Plan (IHP): DIABETES Page 1

Student: _____ D.O.B.: _____ Home Phone: _____

Mother: _____ Work Phone: _____ Cell Phone: _____

Father: _____ Work Phone: _____ Cell Phone: _____

Guardian: _____ Phone: _____

School Nurse: _____ Phone: _____

School: _____ Grade: _____ Teacher: _____

Physician: _____ Phone: _____ Fax: _____

Diabetes Educator: _____ Phone: _____ 504 Plan on file ☐ Yes ☐ No

Hospital of Choice: _____ Date of Diagnosis: _____

Health Concern: Diabetes ☐ Type 1 or ☐ Type 2

Target Blood Glucose Range: _____ to _____

Required blood glucose testing at school: Times to test blood glucose:

☐ Trained personnel must perform blood glucose test.   ☐ Before meals   ☐ Before P.E.   ☐ Other _____

☐ Trained personnel must supervise blood glucose test.   ☐ After meals   ☐ After P.E.

☐ Student can perform testing independently.   ☐ Before snack   ☐ Before getting on bus/going home.

☐ Student can carry supplies and test where needed.   ☐ As needed for signs/symptoms of low/high blood glucose.

Call parent if blood glucose values are below _____ or above _____.

Medications to be given during school hours:

Student is on ☐ oral diabetes medication(s)   Dose: _____ **Times to be given** _____

Student is on ☐ insulin. Type: _____ Dose: _____ **Times to be given** _____

Blood Glucose Correction and Insulin Dosage using (Rapid Acting) Insulin: _____

Blood Glucose Range _____mg/dL (_____ mmol/L) Administer _____ units

Blood Glucose Range _____mg/dL (_____ mmol/L) Administer _____ units

Blood Glucose Range _____mg/dL (_____ mmol/L) Administer _____ units

Blood Glucose Range _____mg/dL (_____ mmol/L) Administer _____ units and check ketones

Blood Glucose Range _____mg/dL (_____ mmol/L) Administer _____ units and check ketones

Blood Glucose Range _____mg/dL (_____ mmol/L) Administer _____ units and check ketones

Blood Glucose Range _____mg/dL (_____ mmol/L) Administer _____ units and check ketones

Insulin to Carbohydrate Ratio _____ unit(s) for every _____ grams of carbohydrate (or to be) eaten

☐ Student independently administers insulin.   ☐ Student self injects with supervision by trained school personnel.

☐ Student self injects with verification of dosage by trained school personnel.

☐ Injections should be done by trained school personnel.

☐ Parent/guardian authorized to increase or decrease sliding scale +/– 2 units of insulin.

☐ Parent/guardian authorized to increase or decrease insulin to carbohydrate count within the following range: 1 unit per prescribed grams of carbohydrates +/– 5 grams of carbohydrates.

Diet: Lunch time: _____ Scheduled P.E. Time: _____ Recess Time: _____

Snack time(s): _____ a.m. _____ p.m.   Location where snacks are kept: _____

Location eaten: _____

Table 2 (continued)
Individualized Health Plan (IHP): DIABETES Page 2

TREATMENT PLAN: Low Blood Glucose (Hypoglycemia) – Below 70 mg/dL (< 3.9 mmol/L)

Causes:

- Too much insulin.
- Too few carbohydrates consumed for the amount of insulin given.
- Too much exercise.
- High excitement.

If you see this:	*Do this:* ACTION PLAN

Signs of Mild Low Blood Glucose (STUDENT IS ALERT)
➤ Headache
➤ Sweating, pale
➤ Shakiness, dizziness
➤ Tired, falling asleep in class
➤ Inability to concentrate
➤ Poor coordination
➤ Other
	1. Have responsible person accompany student to health office or check blood glucose in the classroom.
	2. Check blood glucose.
	3. If less than 70 mg/dL (< 3.9 mmol/L), give one of the following sources of glucose:
	   • 2-4 glucose tablets
	   • 6-9 Sweetarts® candies
	   • 2-4 oz. orange or other 100% juice
	   • 4-6 oz. sugar soda (<u>not sugar-free</u>)
	4. After 15 minutes, check blood glucose again.
	5. Repeat if necessary until blood glucose is > 70 mg/dL

Signs of Moderate Low Blood Glucose (STUDENT IS NOT ALERT)
➤ Severe confusion
➤ Disorientation
➤ Not able to or unwilling to swallow
➤ May be combative
	1. Check blood glucose.
	2. Keeping head elevated, give one of the following forms of glucose:
	   • 1 tube Cake Mate® gel applied between cheek and gum.
	   • ½ - 1 tube instant glucose applied between cheek and gum.
	3. After 15 minutes, check blood glucose again.
	4. Re-treat until blood glucose is > 70 mg/dL (> 3.9 mmol/L).
	5. Notify parent/guardian.

Signs of Severe Low Blood Glucose ➤ Not able or unwilling to swallow ➤ Unconsciousness ➤ Seizure ➤ **GIVE NOTHING BY MOUTH!**	1. Place student on side. 2. If personnel are authorized to use Glucagon, give prescribed dose: _____ mg(s) (Intramuscular or subcutaneous) 3. Call 911, then parent and physician, notify school nurse. 4. Remain with student until help arrives.

Table 2 (continued)
Individualized Health Plan (IHP): DIABETES Page 3

Student: _____ D.O.B.: _____

HIGH BLOOD GLUCOSE:

☐ Student needs to be treated when blood glucose is above _____ mg/dL.

☐ Call parent or guardian when blood glucose is greater than _____ mg/dL.

☐ **Symptoms** could include (check all that apply): ☐ extreme thirst ☐ headache ☐ abdominal pain ☐ nausea ☐ increased urination

Treatment of High Blood Glucose:

✔ Drink 6-16 oz. sugar-free fluids (caffeine free) <u>every hour</u>. ✔ Be allowed to carry water bottle. ✔ Use rest room as often as needed.

☐ Use prescribed sliding scale insulin orders when blood glucose is over _____ mg/dL if no insulin given in past two hours. Recheck blood glucose in two hours.

☐ Check urine ketones or blood ketones, if glucose is greater than **300 mg/dL (> 16.7 mmol/L) 2x** or when ill/and or vomiting.

- If urine ketones are **moderate to large** or if blood ketones are greater than 0.6 mmol/L, **call parent immediately!**
- Recommend child be released from school when ketones are large in order to be treated and monitored more closely by parent/guardian.

✔ **If student exhibits nausea, vomiting, stomacheache or is lethargic, contact parent; student should be released from school.**

✔ **Student can return to class if none of the above physical symptoms are present.**

Field trip information and special events:

1. Notify parent and school nurse in advance so proper training can be accomplished.
2. Adult staff must be trained and responsible for student's needs on field trip.
3. Extra snacks, blood glucose monitor, copy of health plan, glucose gel or other emergency supplies must accompany student on field trip.
4. Adult(s) accompanying student on a field trip will be notified of student's health accommodations on a need to know basis.

SUPPLIES	NEEDED	NOT NEEDED
Blood glucose meter and blood glucose strips	☐	☐
Lancets with lancing device	☐	☐
Blood ketone strips (if using the Precision meter)	☐	☐
Urine ketone strips	☐	☐
Insulin syringes	☐	☐
Antibacterial skin cleanser or alcohol wipes	☐	☐
Bottle of refrigerated rapid acting insulin — Type: _____	☐	☐
Glucose tabs, Cake Mate® gel, juice, or other source of glucose	☐	☐
Carbohydrate snack	☐	☐
Glucogen Emergency Kit®	☐	☐
Sharps container	☐	☐

As parent/guardian of the above named student, I give my permission to the school nurse and other designated staff to perform and carry out the diabetes tasks as outlined in this Individualized Health Plan (IHP) and for my child's healthcare provider to share information with the school nurse for the completion of this plan. I understand that the information contained in this plan will be shared with school staff on a need-to-know basis. It is the responsibility of the parent/guardian to notify the school nurse whenever there is any change in the student's health status or care. I also give the school permission to contact my child's health care provider. Parents/Guardian and student are responsible for maintaining necessary supplies, snacks, blood glucose monitor, medications and equipment.

Parent/Guardian_____ Date_____

School Nurse_____ Date_____

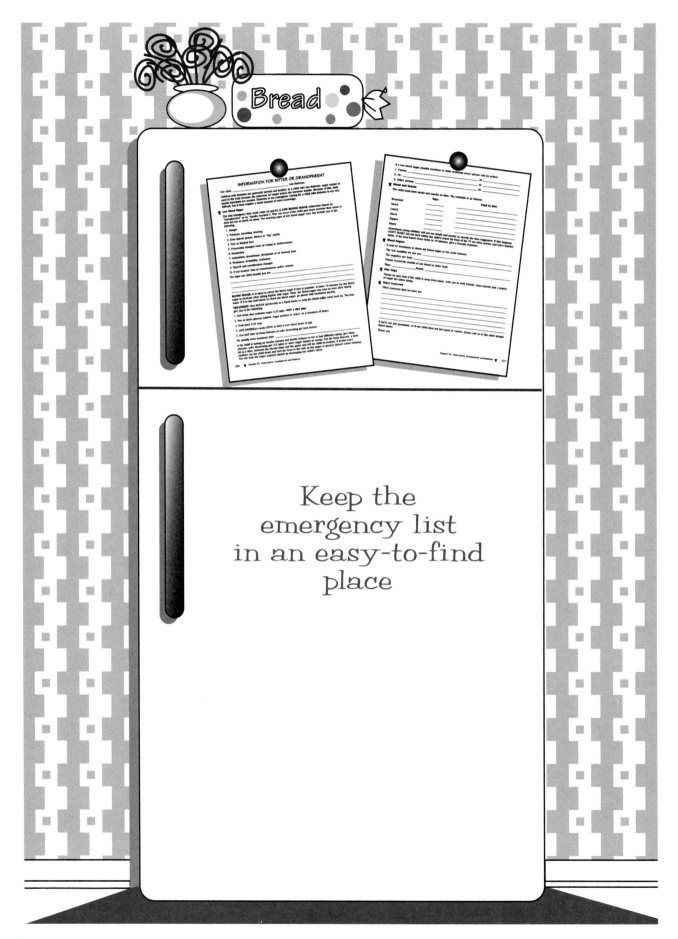

Keep the
emergency list
in an easy-to-find
place

Chapter 26
Child-sitters, Grandparents and Diabetes

It is important for parents to feel that their child is safe with caregivers other than the parents. It is also important for these caregivers to feel confident that they can provide diabetes care.

WHAT DO THEY NEED TO KNOW?

🐾 How much training is needed will depend upon the amount of time the child will be with the caregiver and the age of the child.

All caregivers need:

- some information about signs of low blood sugar and how to treat. A low blood sugar can occur at any time.

- some basic instruction on foods and diabetes. A two-page handout is in this chapter, which can be cut out or copied for the caregiver.

- emergency phone numbers in case the parents cannot be reached. This helps everyone feel better.

- to know how to give shots, when to check for urine or blood ketones, and other more detailed information if the parents are to be away for a longer time period.

- an extra supply of insulin, etc. (in case a bottle is dropped and broken).

🐾 Attending a "Grandparent Workshop" or other workshop can help to teach the grandparents, baby-sitters or other caregivers about diabetes.

- It is important for the child and the grandparents to continue to have a close relationship.

- It can also help to remove any fears about giving shots or treating low blood sugars.

🐾 Caregivers may wish to join the parents at initial education classes or at the time of clinic visits. They are always welcome.

Information for the Sitter or Grandparent

Our child, _____, has diabetes.

Children with diabetes are generally normal and healthy. In a child who has diabetes, sugar cannot be used by the body because the pancreas no longer makes the hormone insulin. Because of this, daily insulin injections are needed. Diabetes is not contagious. Caring for a child with diabetes is not very difficult, but it does require a small amount of extra knowledge.

Low Blood Sugar

The only emergency that could come on quickly is LOW BLOOD SUGAR (otherwise known as "hypoglycemia" or an "insulin reaction"). This can occur if the child gets more exercise than usual or does not eat as much as usual. *The warning signs of low blood sugar vary (see Chapter 6) but may include any of the following:*

1. Hunger
2. Paleness, sweating, shaking
3. Eyes appear glassy, dilated or "big" pupils
4. Pale or flushed face
5. Personality changes such as crying or stubbornness
6. Headaches
7. Inattention, drowsiness, sleepiness at an unusual time
8. Weakness, irritability, confusion
9. Speech and coordination changes
10. If not treated, loss of consciousness and/or seizure

The signs our child usually has are: _____

_____

_____

BLOOD SUGAR: It is ideal to check the blood sugar if this is possible. It takes 10-15 minutes for the blood sugar to increase after taking liquids with sugar. Thus, the blood sugar can even be done after taking sugar. If it is not convenient to check the blood sugar, go ahead with treatment anyway.

TREATMENT: Give SUGAR (preferably in a liquid form) to help the blood sugar rise.

You may give any of the following:

1. One-half cup of soft drink that contains sugar – **NOT a diet pop**
2. Three or four glucose tablets, sugar packets or cubes
3. One-half cup of fruit juice
4. LIFE-SAVERS (FIVE or SIX pieces) or other candy that is less of a choking hazard.
5. One-half tube of Insta-Glucose or cake decorating gel (see below)

We usually treat reactions with: _____

If the child is having a low blood sugar and he/she refuses to eat or has difficulty eating, give Insta-Glucose, cake decorating gel (1/2 tube) or other sugar source. Put the Insta-Glucose, a little bit at a time, between the cheeks (lips) and the gums and tell the child to swallow. If he/she can't swallow, lay the child down and turn the head to the side so the sugar (glucose) doesn't cause choking. You can help the sugar solution absorb by massaging the child's cheek.

If a low blood sugar (insulin reaction) or other problems occur, please call:

1. Parent: _____ at: _____

2. _____ at: _____

3. _____ at: _____

🐾 Meals, Snacks and Insulin

The child must have meals and snacks on time. The schedule is as follows:

	Time	Food to Give	Insulin to Give
Breakfast	_____	_____	_____
Snack	_____	_____	_____
Lunch	_____	_____	_____
Snack	_____	_____	_____
Supper	_____	_____	_____
Snack	_____	_____	_____

Sometimes young children will not eat meals and snacks at exactly the time suggested. If this happens, DON'T PANIC! Set the food within the child's reach (in front of the TV set often works) and leave him/her alone. If the food hasn't been eaten in 10 minutes, give a friendly reminder. Allow about 30 minutes for meals.

🐾 Blood Sugars

It may be necessary to check the blood sugar (Chapter 7) or ketones (Chapter 5).

The supplies we use are: _____

The supplies are kept: _____

Please record the results of any blood sugars or urine ketones in the log book.

Time: _____ Result: _____

🐾 Side Trips

Please be sure that if the child is away from home, with you or with friends, extra snacks and a source of sugar are taken along.

🐾 Other Concerns: *Concerns that we have are:*

_____

_____

_____

_____

_____

If there are any questions or if our child does not feel well or vomits, please call us or the other people listed above. Thank you.

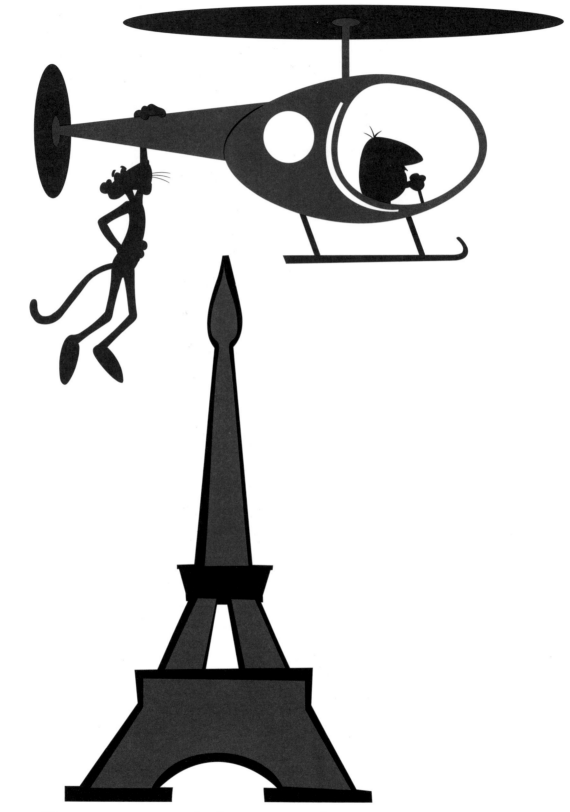

Be prepared for anything when
you're planning to camp or vacation.
Special planning is important for vacations.

Chapter 27
Vacations and Camp

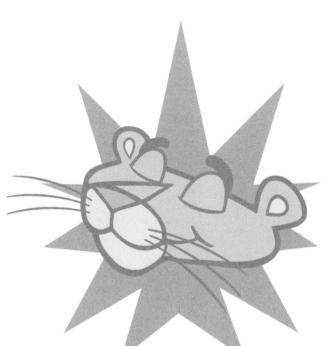

WHEN TRAVELING, WHAT SHOULD PLANNING INCLUDE?

Insulin, blood sugar and ketone strips, glucagon and CGM sensors must be kept in a plastic bag in a cooler if traveling by car. All will spoil if they get above 90° F (32° C) or if they freeze.

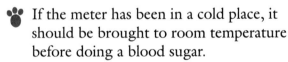 If the meter has been in a cold place, it should be brought to room temperature before doing a blood sugar.

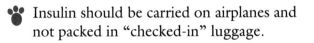 Car travel may result in higher blood/CGM glucose levels due to less activity. Extra insulin is sometimes given.

- Remember to take supplies for measuring ketones.

- Insulin should be carried on airplanes and not packed in "checked-in" luggage.

- Since 9/11/01, it is important with airplane travel to have a vial of insulin with the pre-printed pharmacy label on the outside of the box. The glucagon should also be left in its original container. Carry supplies on-board in case a suitcase is lost. There have been no problems with taking insulin, insulin pumps or other diabetes supplies through security. Insulin pumps

and continuous glucose monitors (CGM) should be worn and not put on the belt (x-ray) or exposed to a body scanner, as electronic components can be altered by x-ray. A letter from the diabetes doctor may also be required (including his/her phone number).

- Extras of everything should be carried by a second person when possible in case one carry-on is lost.

- Extra snacks (sugar [dextrose] tablets, granola bars, etc.) should be carried in case food is late or not available.

- Time changes within the U.S. are usually not a problem, but they must be considered if going overseas (call your doctor or nurse). For insulin pumps, the time in the pump is just reset.

- If traveling by plane and wearing an insulin pump, the high altitude sometimes causes pressure and extra insulin to be administered. Temporary basal rates or discontinuing insulin (maximum of two hours) is sometimes needed.

- If activity is to be increased (playing at the beach, fishing, hiking, going to an amusement park, etc.), the insulin dose should be decreased.

CAMP

• Diabetes camp is often the first chance for a child and parents to show they can survive without each other. Most camps have doctors and nurses present so that the children are safe. Getting to know other children with diabetes who are of a similar age can be very helpful. Most of all, camp should be fun!

• If going to a non-diabetes camp (or school camp/outdoor lab):

- It is essential the camp nurse and cabin counselor know about diabetes (low blood sugars and what to do, high blood sugars and what to do, illness and what to do, etc.).

- Insulin changes for camp will need to be made by the child's diabetes doctor or nurse.

- All diabetes supplies will need to be provided by the family.

- Phone numbers need to be provided to report blood sugars and receive insulin dose changes and for any emergency.

A day at the beach is fun . . .

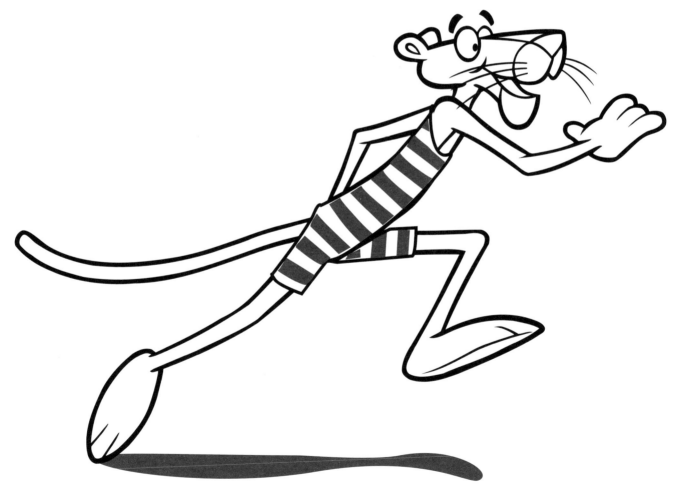

. . . and so is camping.

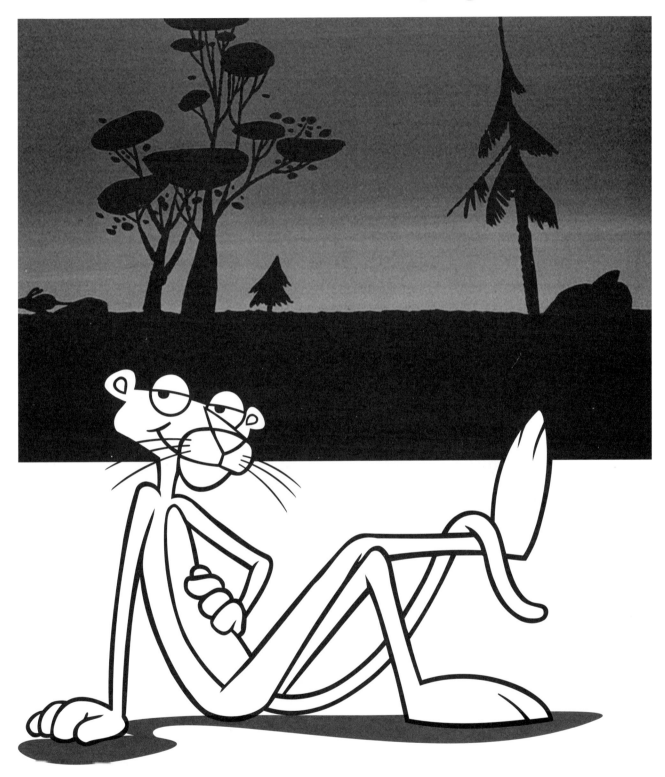

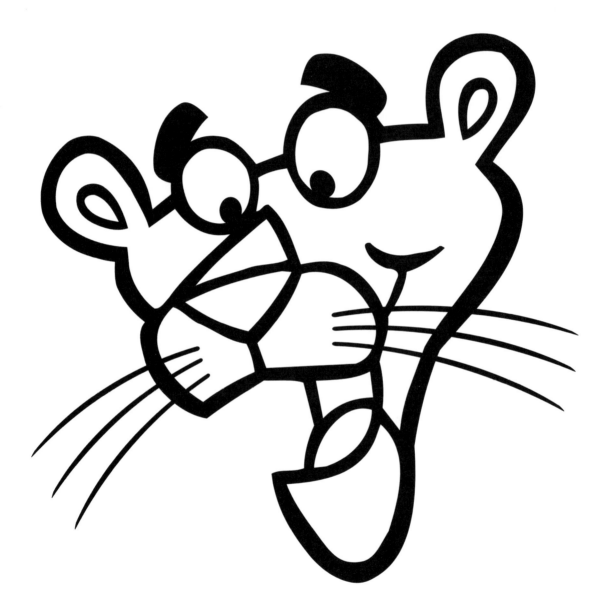

Using an insulin pump
sometimes increases one's energy.

Chapter 28
Insulin Pumps

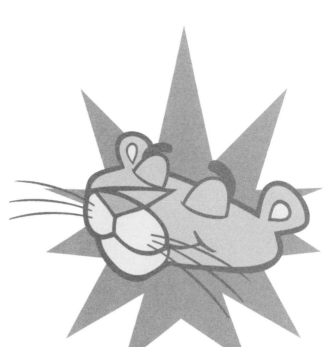

THE PUMP

An insulin pump is a microcomputer (the size of a pager) that constantly provides insulin. It is important to realize that the current insulin pumps do not change the insulin dose administered based on the blood sugar level. Only rapid-acting insulin is used in pumps. Pumps have become more popular in recent years. Advantages and disadvantages of pumps are discussed in Chapter 28 in the larger book, *"Understanding Diabetes"*. In addition, a book *"Understanding Insulin Pumps and Continuous Glucose Monitors"*, is available (see "Ordering Materials" in the back of this book). After reading one or both of these resources, the family may wish to discuss possible pump use with their diabetes care providers.

HOW IS INSULIN GIVEN BY THE PUMP?

 The **basal** dose delivers a preset amount of insulin each hour.

 A **bolus** dose is entered/given by the person wearing the pump (or by an adult) each time food is eaten or if a high blood/CGM glucose level is found.

WHAT IS INVOLVED WHEN STARTING ON A PUMP?

- The first week (and for some, the first month) is the most difficult as the system is learned.

- At least four blood sugars (and/or wearing a continuous glucose monitor [CGM]), must be done each day prior to starting a pump.

- Carbohydrate counting (see Chapter 12) and correction factors (Chapter 22) are used to determine bolus doses.

- Bolus dosages for food are best taken 15-20 minutes before eating (unless the blood/CGM glucose level is low).

- When young children are treated with a pump, the parents are responsible for counting carbohydrates and giving the bolus insulin doses.

- All pumps are now "smart pumps" and have insulin-to-carbohydrate (I/C) ratios and correction factors programmed into them per the physician and family. Then, when a blood sugar and/or grams of carbohydrate to be eaten are entered, the pump suggests an appropriate insulin dose. This dose can be given as suggested or it can be changed.

- Basal and bolus insulin doses are individualized for each person. The physician usually suggests initial basal rates.

- Close contact with the health care providers is essential.

- Our experience shows that children do well if they and their parents are both highly motivated.

- *The person with diabetes must be ready for the pump. It must not be just the parents!*

THREE MAIN PROBLEMS SEEN WITH INSULIN "PUMPERS":

 forgetting to give bolus doses

 getting lazy and not doing at least four blood sugars per day (or consistently wearing a CGM)

the cannula (tube) coming out from under the skin or kinking, causing blood/CGM glucose levels (± ketones) to rapidly rise (remember: only rapid-acting insulin, which is short-lasting, is used in a pump)

THREE ADVANTAGES OF INSULIN PUMPS:

 Insulin dosages can be finely tuned for different periods of the day

 Insulin levels with exercise can be more safely managed

Fewer shots

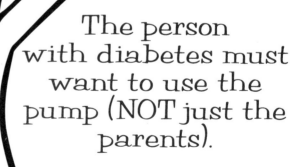

The person with diabetes must want to use the pump (NOT just the parents).

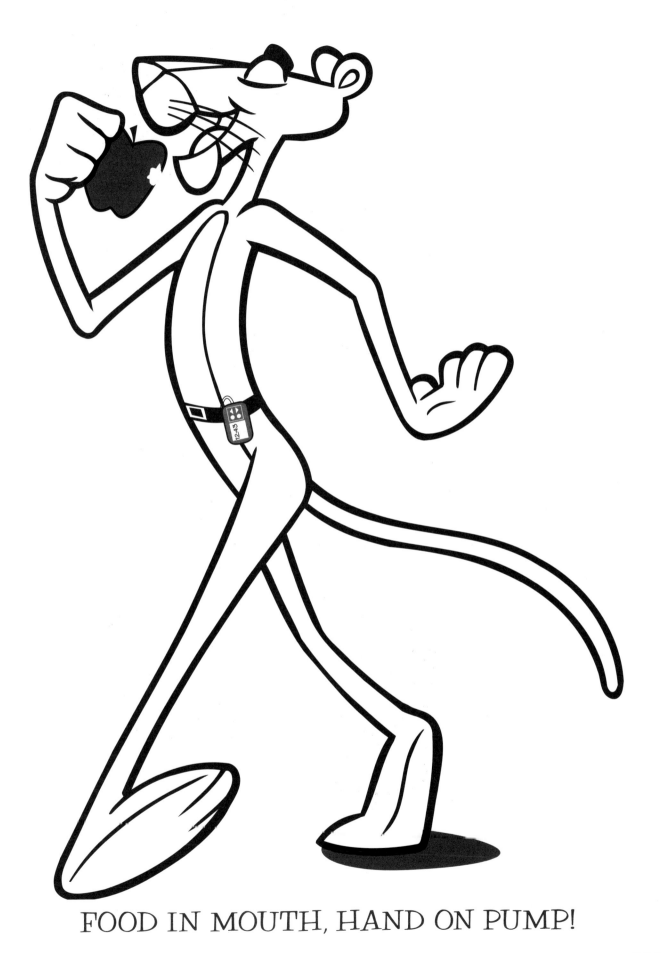

FOOD IN MOUTH, HAND ON PUMP!

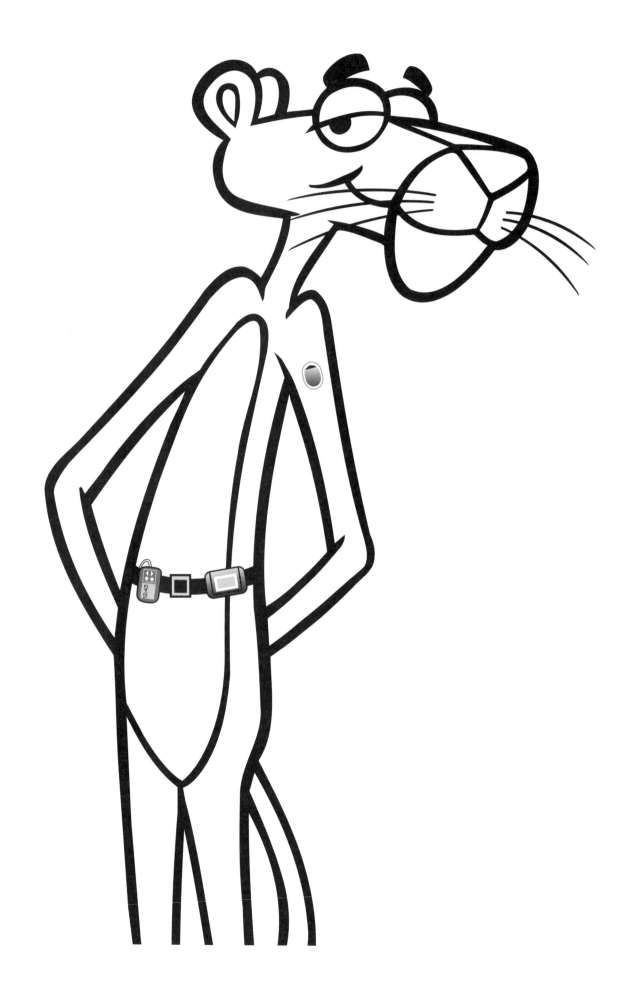

Chapter 29
Continuous Glucose Monitoring (CGM)

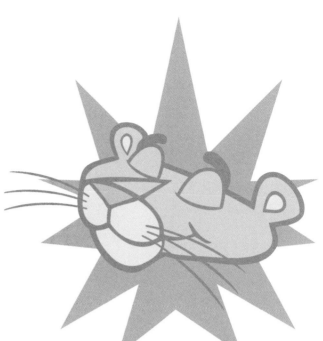

One of the major advances in the treatment of diabetes in recent years has been in the development of continuous glucose monitors (CGM). These devices give readings of subcutaneous (not blood) glucose levels every one to ten minutes. This compares with finger-stick blood sugar (glucose) readings which are usually done only four or five times each day. The subcutaneous CGM glucose values are approximately 10 minutes behind the blood sugar values, as the sugar must pass through the blood vessel wall into the subcutaneous space, and then the CGM system must determine the value. This delay is of almost no clinical significance with the frequency of CGM readings.

The purpose of this chapter is to present a brief overview of CGM. An entire book on Insulin Pumps and CGM is available for people wanting detailed information (*"Understanding Insulin Pumps and Continuous Glucose Monitors"* - see ordering materials in the back of this book). It is important to emphasize that, as with insulin pumps, the CGM technology is not for everyone. Some essential points are:

- The person (except for the very young) and not just the parents must want to use CGM.

- Blood sugar levels must still be done at least twice daily to calibrate the CGM (see below). They must also be done anytime a low blood sugar is suspected and/or the CGM value is in question.

- CGM values will not always match the blood sugar values.

- It usually requires wearing the CGM at least six days per week to have an improved HbA1c value.

THE COMPONENTS OF A CONTINUOUS GLUCOSE MONITOR (CGM)

The CGMs currently available in the US all have three basic parts:

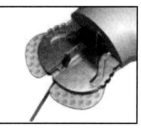

Sensor: As with the insulin pump, a small plastic probe is inserted (with the push of a button) under the skin. The sensor reads subcutaneous (not blood) glucose levels for the next five to seven days (it is often possible to make them last even longer).

Transmitter: The transmitter attaches to the sensor and sends the glucose reading to the receiver.

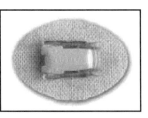

 Receiver or Monitor: The receiver receives the glucose readings from the transmitter

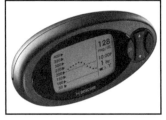

and converts the signal to a level we are used to dealing with for blood sugars. It is a mini computer that records and saves much information. The MiniMed system has the receiver within the insulin pump (for pumpers), but the CGM **DOES NOT** control insulin output by the pump.

INITIATING CGM THERAPY

As with initiation of insulin pump therapy, various clinics will have different protocols. The criteria for deciding who is ready to begin CGM therapy are similar to those discussed for starting an insulin pump.

SOME ADVANTAGES OF CGM

 Glucose levels: Knowing glucose levels every few minutes throughout the day, particularly after meals and during the night, can be a great help.

 Trend graphs: The trend graphs show the direction a glucose level is going (in contrast to a single point in time for a blood sugar level).

 Warning alarms: The alarms for high and low glucose levels can help to prevent episodes of DKA or hypoglycemia.

 Reduced finger pokes: Fewer blood sugars are generally needed.

 Lower HbA1c: If worn consistently (e.g., 6 days per week) HbA1c levels usually decrease.

SOME DIFFICULT ISSUES WITH CGM

There are several areas with which some people/families have difficulty. They are:

 Adhesive issues: Adhesion problem for the sensor/transmitter are one of the two most frequent difficulties with CGM. For some people this goes smoothly and is not a problem. For others, it is a major difficulty. The issues are discussed in detail in the Pump and CGM book.

 Calibration: A second issue with CGM involves calibrating the system so that the CGM values are as accurate as possible and are matching the blood sugar values. Calibration involves doing a finger-stick blood sugar and entering it into the receiver, preferably at a time when the blood sugar is not rapidly changing.

 Alarms: Some people are annoyed by the alarms for high and low glucose levels or for the need to do a calibration. Alarms can be set on "vibrate". If bothersome, discuss with the diabetes care-providers.

 Comfort: The sensors are gradually getting smaller (and more accurate).

 Cost: Insurance coverage should be checked prior to ordering the CGM system. Coverage is gradually improving.

SENSOR PLACEMENT AND ADHESION

Placement: Each CGM company has suggestions for where to place their sensors. In general, they can be worn on the back of the arm, the abdomen, hips, or buttocks. The selected area must have enough skin/fat to be able to pinch up a little bit with two fingers.

Adhesive use: There are many different adhesive wipes, tapes, and bandages that can help sensors to stick to skin. It is quite common for a person to use an adhesive wipe to treat the skin under the sensor, to then place the sensor on the skin, and finally to reinforce it with additional tape. Every person is different, and what works for one person may not work for others. Detailed suggestions are given in the Pump and CGM book.

CGM DATA

There are two main types of data that can be obtained from CGM usage: **Real-Time and Retrospective**. Real-time data refers to data available while wearing the CGM (such as a "trend-graph" showing a series of glucose values). Retrospective data refers to data from the past-most often downloaded using a computer. Both types of data are important and are explained in detail in the Pump and CGM book.

In summary, CGM use is not for everyone. However, when ready and willing, the CGM can provide additional information as well as safety.

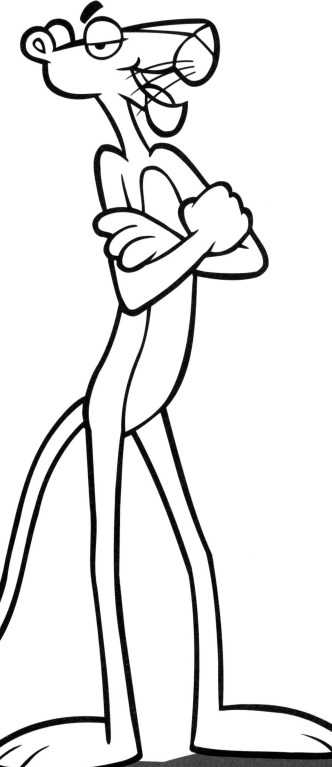

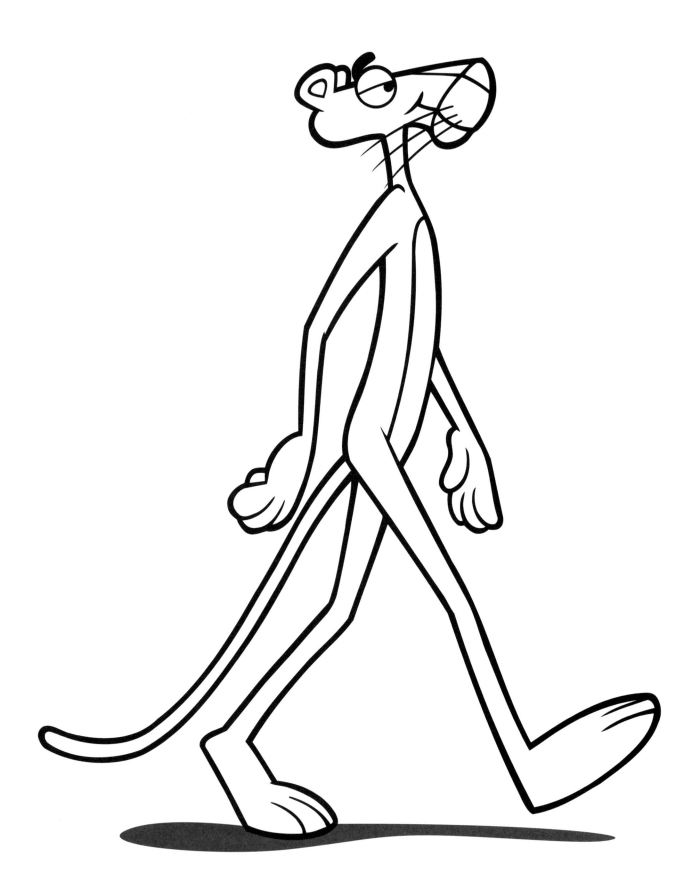

Good sugar control prior to pregnancy
is essential!

110

Chapter 30

Pregnancy and Diabetes

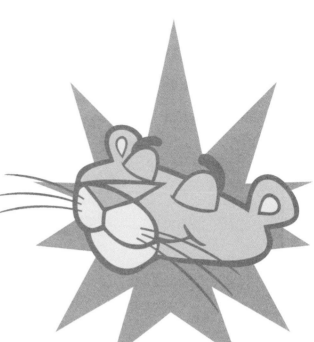

Pregnancy is possible for women with diabetes who do not have severe problems with complications.

WHAT IS IMPORTANT WHEN THINKING ABOUT GETTING PREGNANT?

 Pregnancy should be <u>planned</u>.

 The best sugar control possible should be achieved before and during pregnancy. The HbA1c should be below 6.5 percent.

 The risk of a miscarriage as well as birth defects in the baby are less if blood sugar/CGM values are normal or near normal when the pregnancy begins.

 Folic acid should be taken for three months before the pregnancy to also help prevent birth defects.

HOW CAN THE BEST SUGAR CONTROL BE ACHIEVED?

 Intensive insulin therapy is usual during pregnancy. This includes:

- an insulin pump or frequent insulin shots

- frequent blood sugar checks (eight to ten a day) or CGM

- paying close attention to nutrition

- frequent contact with the healthcare team

 The target values for blood sugar/CGM values are lower than usual and are given in the table in Chapter 30 of *"Understanding Diabetes"*.

 Clinic visits are also more often: usually every two to four weeks.

WHAT ABOUT COMPLICATIONS AND PREGNANCY?

 Kidney damage is usually not a problem during pregnancy unless already present before the pregnancy. Medicines used to prevent kidney damage called "ACE-inhibitors" should not be taken during pregnancy. This medicine could cause birth defects in the baby.

 The eyes should be checked more often during pregnancy (at least every three months). If moderate damage is already present, this may get worse during pregnancy.

GESTATIONAL DIABETES

- Gestational diabetes is diabetes that develops as a result of the stress of the pregnancy. Regular exercise and diet are important.

  - After diagnosis, the care is similar to that of a person who had diabetes prior to pregnancy.

  - Gestational diabetes usually goes away after pregnancy. There is an increased risk of developing type 2 diabetes later in life.

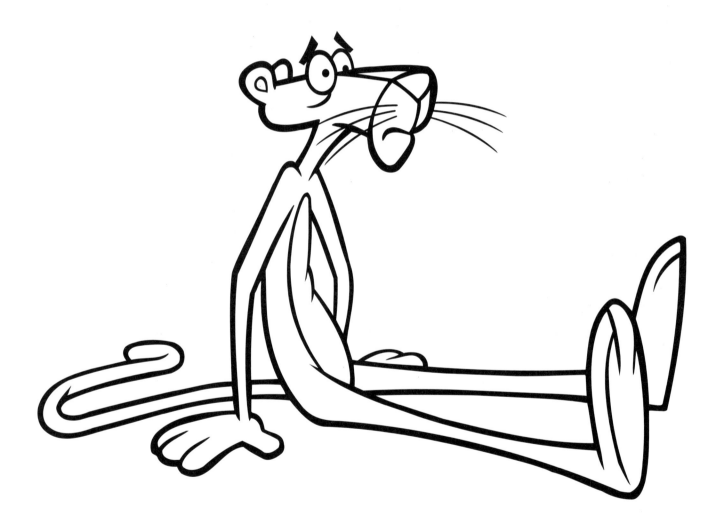

Chapter 31

Research and Diabetes

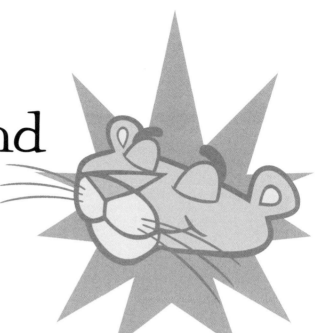

This area is always changing.

THE FIVE SUBJECTS PEOPLE ASK MOST ABOUT ARE:

 A Cure:

Pancreas or islet transplantation is already possible. The problem is that the strong medicines necessary to prevent rejection can be more harmful than having diabetes. Many new medicines are being tried, but it is still early. Fortunately, advances are being made in the intensive management of diabetes, providing this as an alternative to surgical transplantation and a life of immunosuppression.

 A "Bionic" Pancreas:

The term "bionic" pancreas refers to a continuous glucose monitor (CGM) sending glucose data to a mini computer which then instructs an insulin pump to give more or less insulin. It is likely that they will become available with one function at a time. Because severe hypoglycemia is dangerous, the ability to turn off an insulin pump with a low glucose value, or a predicted low glucose

level, will likely be approved first. Other features, such as glucose control during the night, will then gradually be added.

A book, "*Understanding Insulin Pumps and Continuous Glucose Monitors*" is now available (see "Ordering Materials" in the back of this book).

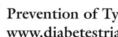 **Prevention of Type 1 Diabetes (see www.diabetestrialnet.org):**

- Several trials are currently under way.

- In the U.S., people can call 1-800-425-8361 to find out where to go for a free TrialNet antibody screening. This area is moving very rapidly.

- Four biochemical islet cell antibodies (Chapter 3) are being used to determine if the autoimmune process has begun. If it has, research trials are enrolling people in studies to try to reverse the process and prevent diabetes.

- Prevention trials are now focused on:

  ~ preventing the autoimmune process from starting

  ~ reversing the autoimmune process to prevent diabetes

  ~ stopping further damage to the islets after diabetes has been diagnosed

- It is likely that prevention will come before a safe cure.

 Prevention of Type 2 Diabetes:

- This has already been shown to be possible.

- It involves eating less, exercising more, and losing weight.

- It is discussed in Chapter 4 of *"Understanding Diabetes"*.

 Prevention of Complications:

- Diabetes complications of the eyes and kidneys are decreasing through attention being paid to the following:

  ~ better sugar control

  ~ exercise and a healthy diet

~ blood pressure control

~ not smoking

~ yearly eye exams and urine microalbumin levels (to check the kidneys). These are essential after three years of diabetes in people age 12 years or older (see Chapter 23). Families may need to help remind their diabetes care provider to make sure these are done each year.

Finding the cure

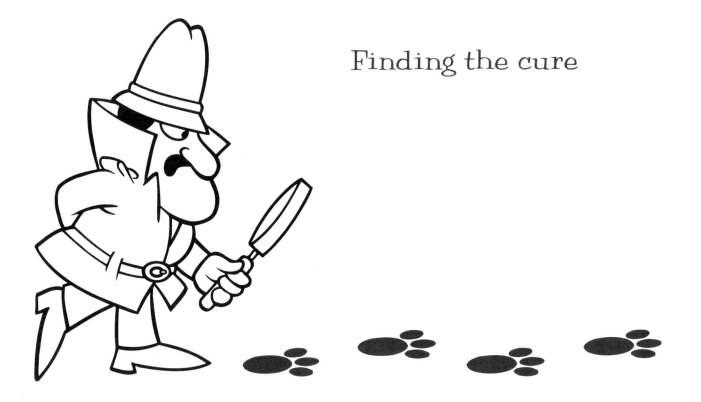

Continuous Glucose Monitoring (CGM) is here!

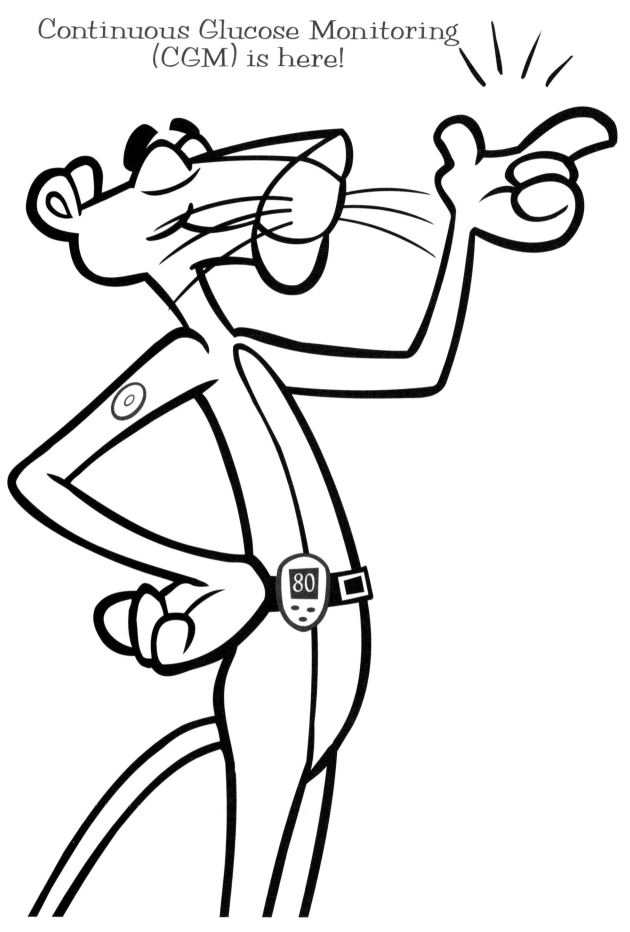

Someday there will be
A CURE FOR DIABETES!

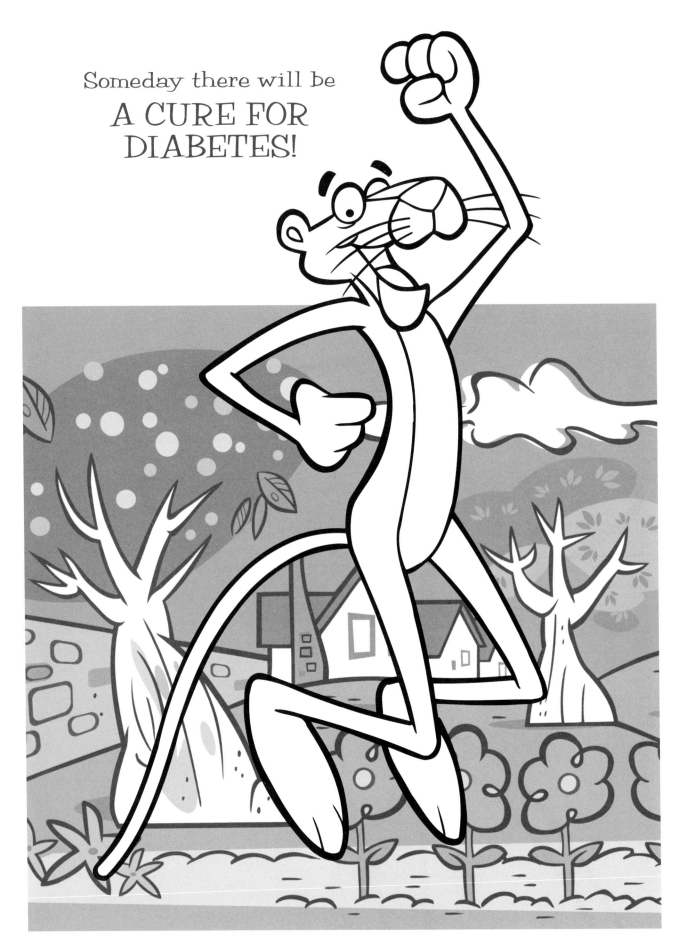

ORDERING MATERIALS

Additional copies of *A First Book for Understanding Diabetes* as well as other diabetes informational material may be ordered by using this form, by calling the Children's Diabetes Foundation at 303-863-1200 or 800-695-2873, or by visiting our website at www.ChildrensDiabetesFoundation.org

Children's Diabetes Foundation

4380 South Syracuse Street • Suite 430 • Denver, CO 80237

Name: _____

Address: _____

City, State, ZIP: _____

Phone: _____ Email: _____

Quantity	Item	Price	Total
	A First Book for Understanding Diabetes Presents the essentials from Understanding Diabetes in synopsis-fashion	$12.00*	
	Un Primer Libro Para Entender La Diabetes Spanish version of ***A First Book for Understanding Diabetes***	$10.00*	
	Understanding Diabetes – "The Pink Panther Book" 12th Edition	$20.00*	
	Understanding Insulin Pumps and Continuous Glucose Monitors Second Edition	$18.00*	
	Diabetes: A History of a Center and a Patient Our newest book, covering the history of the Barbara Davis Center for Childhood Diabetes and following a fictitious patient's concerns and struggles with the disease.	$15.00*	
	SHIPPING AND HANDLING: $5.00 per book for orders of 1-9 books $2.00 per book for orders of 10 books and over	Shipping and Handling	
		TOTAL	

*Prices subject to change.

❏ Please include me on the Children's Diabetes Foundation mailing list.

❏ Check enclosed payable to: Children's Diabetes Foundation

❏ VISA   ❏ MasterCard   ❏ Discover   ❏ AmEx

Card # _____ Exp. Date _____

All orders must be paid in full before delivery. Books are mailed USPS or Ground UPS. Allow one to three weeks for delivery.

Canadian and Foreign Purchasers: Please include sufficient funds to equal U.S. currency exchange rates.

For quantity order pricing and additional information call 303-863-1200 or 800-695-2873 or visit our website at www.ChildrensDiabetesFoundation.org

WEBSITES

Barbara Davis Center for Childhood Diabetes
University of Colorado Denver
Mail Stop A140
P.O. Box 6511
Aurora, CO 80045
303-724-2323 · Fax 303-724-6779
www.BarbaraDavisCenter.org

Children's Diabetes Foundation at Denver, Colorado
www.ChildrensDiabetesFdn.org

Children With Diabetes
www.ChildrenwithDiabetes.com

Juvenile Diabetes Research Foundation
www.jdrf.org

American Diabetes Association
www.diabetes.org